"To begin on an unequivocal note, let it be understood that Dr. Mintz has shined a bright light on a fragmented healthcare delivery system for autistic individuals that is ineffective, inconsistent, and improvident beyond belief. However, through a series of poignant stories, made possible by medical and behavioral science, Dr. Mintz demonstrates the power of a holistic, integrated medical home for autism treatment. His model of care clearly produces the coveted trinity of outcomes: capability, comfort, and calmness for his patients. *Optimizing Outcomes* may well be considered the harbinger of hope for families, and a blueprint for professionals."

MICHAEL J. CAMERON, Ph.D., BCBA-D,
LBA, University of Southern California

"Our son Matthew suffered from recurring bouts of vomiting from the time he was six months old. In search of a cure, we had taken him to every specialist in every world-renowned medical facility we could find. He underwent more medical testing than any small child should ever have to endure, yet no one could give us answers. And then our world changed when we met Dr. Mintz at NeurAbilities Healthcare. After our first visit with Dr. Mintz, we left with a treatment plan and Matt never had an episode again. It is my hope that by telling Matt's story, and other stories from families like ours, we can save a family from the six years of suffering we endured. As Matt's mom, I know Dr. Mintz saved Matt's life."

JENNIFER WILLIAMS, Matt's grateful mom

T0143839

"Dr. Mark Mintz's vision of integrated health care for families dealing with neurodevelopmental disability grew into a reality, step-by-step, over three decades. *Optimizing Outcomes* describes the process of creating a novel health care model—identifying the need, understanding the complexity, developing the mission, coordinating the resources, applying the neuroscience, and optimizing the outcomes. Dr. Mintz is a true visionary with compassion as well as a master team-builder who knows how to implement ideas into interdisciplinary and comprehensive clinical care. An amazing narrative about a creative means to a better end."

WILLIAM D. GRAF, MD, Child Neurologist; Professor of
Pediatrics, University of Connecticut School of Medicine

"*Optimizing Outcomes* is so well written you can feel the emotion of what the people Dr. Mintz writes about are experiencing, and the impact their health is having on their lives. *Optimizing Outcomes* gives hope that, with the help of Specialty Care Medical Home practices, children with autism need not be 'defined by their diagnosis,' but it will only be a part of who they are. People can get the help that they need."

LIZA GUNDELL, CEO, Autism Family Services of New Jersey

"I encourage both health care professionals, caregivers, and the public to read Dr. Mark Mintz's significant contributions in *Optimizing Outcomes* describing and proposing innovative healthcare delivery models for the underserved population of special needs individuals. Readers will find essential information and guidance for developing solutions for improving the lives of those suffering from both common and complex Neurodevelopmental Disabilities."

JAMES M. OLESKE, MD, MPH, François-Xavier
Bagnoud Distinguished Professor of Pediatrics-
Emeritus, Rutgers - New Jersey Medical School

"In working with Dr. Mark Mintz, I have had the privilege to see firsthand how he has literally changed the world for so many children with neurobehavioral disorders and provided hope to their very distraught families. His book, *Optimizing Outcomes,* is a compelling read in which you will learn that he is an extraordinary physician who successfully diagnoses and treats children who have been failed by our healthcare system. You will come to understand his powerful vision and innovative solution for delivering care to the special needs population that is growing in staggering numbers year after year."

TONI PERGOLIN, President and CEO, Bancroft

"The nervous system is typically treated by the medical profession as if its problems are either neurology, psychiatry, or psychology. There is no clean separation, however, for neurobehavioral problems. *Optimizing Outcomes* describes how to heal this artificial rift using a unified 'specialty care medical home' approach that is coordinated and more effective."

MICHAEL SEGAL, MD, PhD,
Founder and Chief Scientist, SimulConsult

"An inspiring and thought-provoking book chronicling the journey of a child neurologist's pursuit of innovative healthcare delivery for individuals with neurodevelopmental and intellectual disabilities. This multifaceted story is a testament to the power of science, ethics, and evidence-based ideas in shaping the future of healthcare. The author's passion and dedication to his craft shines through in the development of a groundbreaking medical home model, recognized with an award from the American Academy of Neurology in 2023. This specialty care medical home model utilizing personalized, precision medical approaches is truly a "one-stop-shop" for compassionate and excellent healthcare delivery. Patients, parents, caregivers, stakeholders, and policymakers alike will find *Optimizing Outcomes* to be a must-read in the search for new cost-effective healthcare systems for complex special needs populations. Overall, this book is an invaluable resource for anyone seeking to improve outcomes and continuity of care for individuals with neurological, neurodevelopmental, and intellectual disabilities."

MARCIO LEYSER, MD, MSc, PhD, Professor of
Pediatrics/Developmental and Behavioral Pediatrics,
University of Iowa Carver College of Medicine

OPTIMIZING
OUTCOMES

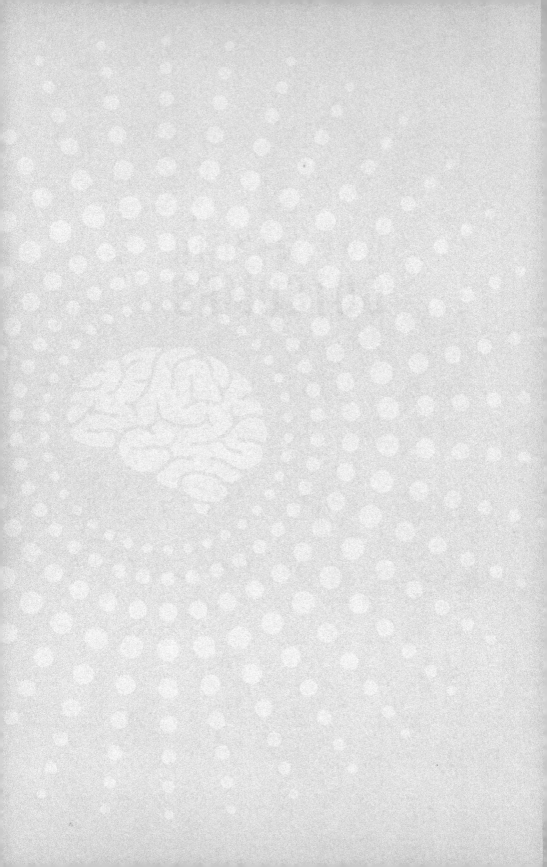

OPTIMIZING
OUTCOMES

Integrated Specialty Healthcare
for Individuals with
Neurodevelopmental Disabilities

MARK MINTZ, M.D.

Advantage | Books

Published by Advantage, Charleston, South Carolina.
Member of Advantage Media.

ADVANTAGE is a registered trademark, and the Advantage colophon is a trademark of Advantage Media Group, Inc.

Printed in the United States of America.

10 9 8 7 6 5 4 3 2 1

ISBN: 978-1-64225-544-7 (Paperback)
ISBN: 978-1-64225-543-0 (eBook)

Library of Congress Control Number: 2023905816

Cover design by Hampton Lamoureux.
Layout design by Lance Buckley.

This publication is designed to provide accurate and authoritative information in regard to the subject matter covered. It is sold with the understanding that the publisher is not engaged in rendering legal, accounting, or other professional services. If legal advice or other expert assistance is required, the services of a competent professional person should be sought.

Advantage Media helps busy entrepreneurs, CEOs, and leaders write and publish a book to grow their business and become the authority in their field. Advantage authors comprise an exclusive community of industry professionals, idea-makers, and thought leaders. Do you have a book idea or manuscript for consideration? We would love to hear from you at **AdvantageMedia.com**.

This book is dedicated to the memory of my father, Dr. Morris Y. Mintz, a World War II veteran, pharmacist, and family physician, who inspired and taught me the importance of the physician-patient relationship in clinical medicine and the value of an extraordinary work ethic empowering a fulfilling life of service.

And to my mother, Sally, who always believed in me, had faith in my abilities, supported my ideas, and trusted my instincts.

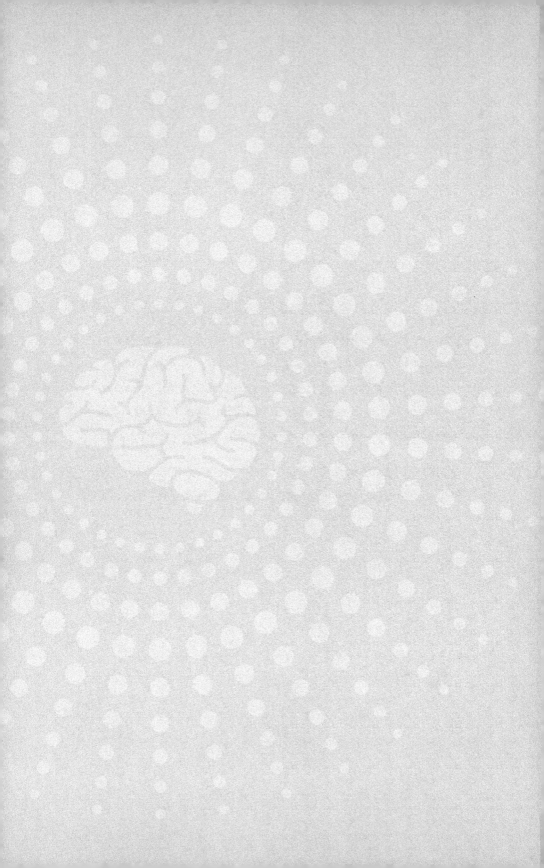

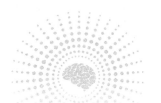

C O N T E N T S

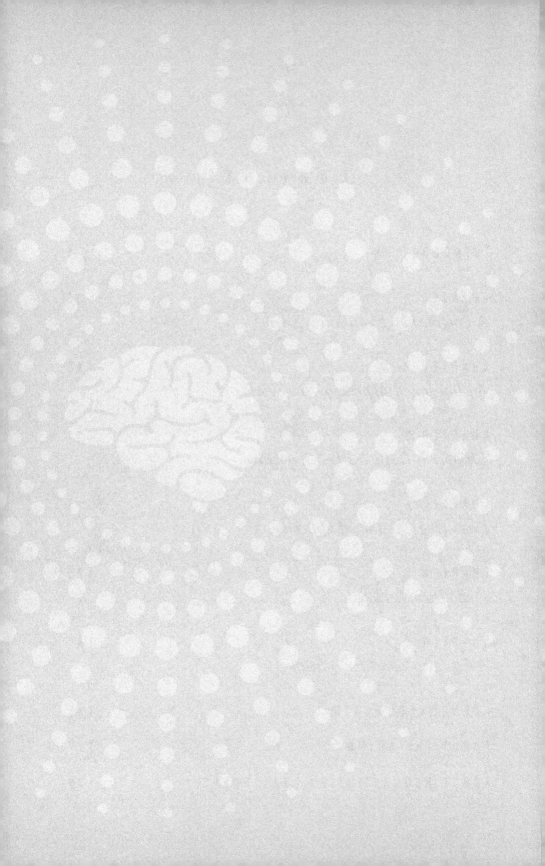

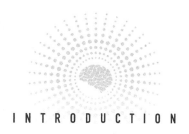

The mother of a three-year-old boy was told she should accept that her son was going to end up institutionalized. This doom-filled prophecy was given by a hospital-based healthcare professional, a clinician. But it was easy to see why.

At three, Michael (not his real name) had no language, and thus, he communicated his fear and pain with physical violence. He was a terror. In a household with older twin siblings, Michael had turned his family's once-peaceful home life into strife-filled chaos by literally and figuratively bouncing off walls and swinging from the curtains every chance he got. Anyone who attempted to corral him would receive a sure reward: a fist to the face. The household was in crisis. The twins were traumatized, and his mother was on the verge of an emotional breakdown twenty-four hours a day.

Imagine the dream every couple has when they bring children into their lives, the beautiful fantasy they weave for the future. Whether it entails a swing set in the backyard, snuggling on the couch in front of a movie, soccer games, or music lessons—whatever it is, every family starts with a dream.

In this case, this couple's vision for a happy family life had been utterly shattered.

But Michael's mother was not ready to give up; indeed, the challenge fueled her. She is one of those parents who, in the very best sense, refuses to take no for an answer. She would not accept the perceived inevitable. She was prepared to achieve the impossible; the only variables for her were how much work it would take and how long. People like Michael's mother are the ones who often find their way through our doors.

Against all odds, Michael's mother undertook the herculean task of personally coordinating and overseeing services for her son in a complex, disjointed, expensive healthcare system. She understood quickly that the system of delivering care to a child with disabilities was the obstacle course she would have to navigate.

Michael's mother and her troubled son found their way to the healthcare organization founded by my wife, Pnina, and me, The Center for Neurological and Neurodevelopmental Health (CNNH), the precursor to NeurAbilities Healthcare, which was even then establishing itself in the healthcare field for an innovative interdisciplinary model of evidence-based intervention for the evaluation and treatment of autism and other neurodevelopmental and neurological disorders.

I began my medical career in the 1980s as a pediatric neurologist serving with the US Public Health Service—National Health Service Corps on assignment to Newark, New Jersey, which was experiencing an epidemic of pediatric patients suffering from the effects of a deadly novel virus of the time—the human immunodeficiency virus (HIV). In that role, I observed the difficulty many clinicians were having recognizing the traumatic impact of acquired immunodeficiency syndrome (AIDS) on patients' neurological and cognitive functions ("NeuroAIDS"), as well as the psychosocial welfare of patients and their families.

I was unaware of it at the time, but the valuable experiences and lessons learned from evaluating and treating NeuroAIDS would be applicable to developing healthcare delivery models and treatment services for those with autism and related disorders. Focusing on neurological disorders in children and bumping up against the same systemic challenges in the healthcare system prompted Pnina and me to open our own healthcare organization, then called The Center for Neurological and Neurodevelopmental Health, or CNNH, now called NeurAbilities Healthcare.

As past president and chief executive officer of CNNH for the first fourteen years and presently chief medical officer of NeurAbilities Healthcare, I and my colleagues continue to develop the robust multidisciplinary "Specialty Care Medical Home" model that I had first conceptualized at Bancroft (a nonprofit provider of programs and services for individuals with autism, those who have intellectual and developmental disabilities, and those in need of neurological rehabilitation, based in Mt. Laurel, New Jersey), where I had served as executive medical director.

By the time Michael came to visit our medical center, following the evolution of our proprietary clinical model in the treatment of autism spectrum disorders, I recommended that the family seek applied behavior analysis (ABA), which is empirically proven to be the most effective behavioral treatment for autism spectrum disorder.

If you had seen Michael when he was a preschooler, you would understand his mother's commitment and intensity. Our staff doted on him and described him as a sweet child with giant sapphire eyes. They commented on how he loved to cuddle with his mom and eat bologna and butter sandwiches. In the rare moments in which he seemed to be at peace, he ignited our own intensity to help turn his life around. We are motivated to help unlock the potential of every child we serve, irrespective of their situation, but seeing the dedication of his family provided additional inspiration.

From ages three to five, Michael received intensive treatment fourteen hours a day for his problematic behaviors and communication and social skill impairments: the core deficits of autism.

With his mother engaged in the full-time job as "traffic controller" among an array of practitioners that included a neuropsychologist, a speech therapist, and occupational and physical therapists, and with continued neurological visits to us for treatment of attention deficits, Michael made rapid progress. He went to school and performed well, scoring grades in the top 2 percent of all the children in his grade.

Defying original prognoses, Michael became an honor student attending a mainstream high school in Philadelphia. Although Michael has communicated with his peers regarding his autism diagnosis, he is indistinguishable from his teenage counterparts and is maturing into a healthy, happy, and funny young man. Michael still has autism, but he is independent in advocating for himself and his needs. Far from being institutionalized, he manages his autism with therapy, medication, and other supports and is forging a life of independence. Michael would say he is not defined by his diagnosis; it is one part of him that he must master in order to flourish.

How is this dramatic success story possible? Michael's mother made two critical decisions to ensure his future. First, she sought early and intensive intervention for his autism. Numerous studies have demonstrated that the earlier children begin their treatment, the better the long-term outcomes. During the preschool years, a child's brain is at its most "plastic," which maximizes the opportunity to develop new neural pathways that facilitate rapid learning. Diagnosing Michael as early as possible and seeking treatment promptly were vital steps in his extraordinary development.[1]

The other significant component was his mother's refusal to accept conventional American healthcare system methods, which

---

1   Wendy L. Stone and Theresa Foy DiGeromino, "There Is No Debate or Doubt: Early Intervention Is Your Child's Best Hope for the Future," UNC Autism Research Center, University of North Carolina–Chapel Hill, accessed March 9, 2023, https://autism. unc.edu/resources/early-intervention.

historically have been focused on improving outcomes of medical diseases, with fewer resources devoted to neuropsychiatric and neurobehavioral (commonly referred to as "mental health") disorders. Her willingness to spend the time relentlessly jousting with every element of the system, including insurers, public education, siloed healthcare providers and more, and to find providers who understood the need to integrate their services and fill the gaps in diagnosis and treatment, optimized Michael's opportunity to achieve success in developing cognitive, social, and developmental functions.

We should be careful here to note that children with autism are never "cured," although a minority can "recover." Because autism has a biological origin, autistic children's brains work differently than neurotypical children's brains, and they will continue to work differently as adults. Many of the behaviors and pathologies associated with autism that impede independent adult functioning can be controlled and even eliminated through treatment, though many associated conditions involving neurological, psychological, and physiological challenges may remain.

This book is about our story of bridging the gaps in the currently fragmented system of care for patients with autism spectrum disorders and other neurodevelopmental disabilities while adhering to precision and evidence-based medical sciences. It is the story of our unique "Specialty Care Medical Home" model for healthcare delivery for special-needs populations: an independent, empirically based, holistic, interdisciplinary, and transdisciplinary approach that has delivered improved outcomes and qualities of life for patients and their families. It is our diagnosis of the problem and our prescription for a solution.

It is a road map for hope.

But first, let's start with how we got here. Let's discuss three issues in the American healthcare system today that bear heavy responsibility for the waste and suboptimal outcomes it produces for patients.

GAPS IN THE SYSTEM

My realization that gaps in the healthcare system are distorting how care is delivered and funded began early in my career when I observed a series of dots that were not being connected. It hearkens back to the early days of the HIV/AIDS epidemic when no one could understand why infants and children were succumbing to confounding opportunistic infections previously unseen at that age and developing mysterious neurological degenerative disorders.

Others in our organization came to the same realization in different ways. For example, our behavioral therapists report that the disconnect between their disciplines and the medical community's approaches in the treatment of children with autism spectrum disorders led to fragmented treatment that failed to capitalize on a variety of perspectives and types of expertise.

THE OVERUSE OF MEDICATION

Our present healthcare system tends toward the study and treatment of disease and only more recently has shifted into preservation and maintenance of health and prevention of disease. This has led to a reliance on pharmacological solutions and interventions to various medical and behavioral conditions and disorders. Particularly in the realm of behavioral healthcare, the reflex is less to understand the cause of symptoms than to suppress them, usually with medication.

In this model, if the medication fails, the antidote is, usually, more or different medication, until all forms of drugs are exhausted—with far less effort and time spent on understanding biological or environmental causes or mechanisms of adverse behavioral manifestations. Although such an approach can be successful, it is not necessarily sustainable and often fraught with short-term and long-term medication side effects and adverse events. Understanding the biological and other causes and contributions to neurological, neurodevelopmental, and neurobehavioral disorders leads to treatments targeted at mechanisms of disease, improves outcomes and quality of life, and reduces reliance on or eliminates pharmacological interventions.

We see and hear examples of this all the time, and I will document them in this book. They remind us that prescribing medication is the easiest course of action in response to a health condition but cannot substitute for understanding its underlying causes. Pharmacological efficacy depends on the difficult detective work of targeting the biological causative source, and too often, it is employed as a shorthand for suppressing symptoms. The adverse impact on patients is staggering.

OVERUTILIZATION OF RESOURCES AND FINANCIAL WASTE

We are on a mission to revamp the delivery of specialized healthcare services to thousands of patients in desperate need of the kinds of care we provide, boost outcomes, and slash costs for the benefit of children, their families, and the communities around them.

Widening the lenses of service providers and insurance companies to include all the natural environments in which children with autism live beyond the therapy room or doctors' offices will lead to better diagnoses and more informed treatment regimens.

Later in the book, one of our patients, Bobbi, enthusiastically tells the story of her tortured journey through America's disjointed healthcare system. Bobbi's decade-long diagnostic odyssey caused her needless pain and suffering, and cost the healthcare system (i.e., all consumers of healthcare) hundreds of thousands, and perhaps even millions, of dollars. In the end, one of our astute neurologists did a few simple and inexpensive tests that revealed a genetic defect and informed us about a safe, low-cost medication that eliminated her symptoms and recurrent hospitalizations.

Bobbi's story is dramatic but not particularly unusual in our current healthcare system. Her experience, particularly her diagnostic odyssey, can be minimized by employing more independent, interdisciplinary specialty care enterprises like ours. Unfortunately, tragically few exist, and the barriers to entry are significant.

Disentangling services from hospitals and medical schools, where they compete with corporate priorities and are strangled by bureaucratic red tape, and establishing them in independent operations akin to ours can break down the silos and help healthcare professionals focus instead on finding solutions for these populations with special needs.

SCALING UP OUR SOLUTIONS

Any organization providing a service desperately needed by significant numbers of people is bound to grow. For example, many high-tech companies providing search engines may owe their success to a variety of factors, including smart management, but the primary impetus behind their growth is that their technologies can answer our questions in a fraction of a second, billions of times every day. These tech companies are filling a need—and doing it very well.

Although we are not a high-tech megacompany, our enterprise has been able to achieve success. From its founding in the years prior to the Great Recession of 2008 to the 2018 inflection point when we brought on investors, our company had grown tenfold without any outside investment simply because we listened to and answered questions plaguing families of children with autism spectrum disorders and other neurological issues. A team of physicians, clinicians, and scientists reinforcing each other's expertise and sharing myriad perspectives for the good of their patients has resonated with people throughout our initial catchment area of greater Philadelphia and New Jersey.

People like Bobbi and Michael's mother and hundreds of others have made their way to us, often after a series of traumatic experiences and diagnostic odysseys, because we have a formula for delivering healthcare services that they need. Our independence allows us to remain nimble and quickly adapt to change, as we did in response to the COVID-19 crisis.

Our organization has been driven by maintaining a laser focus on our vision and mission, which has been validated by our dramatic growth despite many challenges and tribulations, including a severe recession in 2008 soon after our formation.

Why should a start-up organization like ours survive and flourish in the shadow of some of the finest medical institutions in the country and, for the first fourteen years, without outside investment?

We have succeeded because we addressed the gaps in healthcare delivery for special needs populations and created a healthcare delivery system that fills these shortcomings. And an independence that frees us from institutional bureaucracies and agendas allows us to work with, rather than for, hospitals and other healthcare institutions. Ultimately, the best of intentions and efforts would be meaningless if we are unable to improve the lives of those who seek our services, often desperately. The experiences and outcomes of people like Bobbi and Michael's mother and thousands of others we have had the privilege to serve make it all worthwhile, authenticating our vision and mission.

Our independence was also a hindrance to business growth. We lacked the leverage to negotiate with payers or the ability to invest in necessary information technology (IT) systems and fulfill electronic medical records (EMR) requirements. The healthcare regulatory framework grew more complex over the years and started placing strain on our management team. The combination of these challenges constrained our ability to serve all the patients who needed us.

In an area of the country where autism spectrum disorder is even more prevalent—now one in thirty-five children in New Jersey[2]—the demand is growing ever faster. Disappointed that we were unable to help all the families who needed our services, we decided it was imperative that we grow exponentially rather than incrementally, as we had done over the previous fourteen years. Being committed to helping all families and children with autism spectrum disorders and other neurological conditions means, for us, providing our unique services to as many of them as possible. That means more clinicians, more services, more administrators, and more investors sharing the risk.

We have helped so many people over the years who would not have reached the level they did without our help. Everyone in the communities we serve should have that opportunity.

We recognized that we could not cross that Rubicon without a bridge. The gap was too wide, and our resources were too meager. At the same time, we knew we had something special—a vision and operating practices that challenge much of the conventional wisdom of the healthcare system—and we were not willing to endanger that with an ill-conceived arrangement. This was not to be cashing in or selling out; it was to be rocket fuel for our liftoff.

2   M. J. Maenner et al., "Prevalence and Characteristics of Autism Spectrum Disorder among Children Aged 8 Years — Autism and Developmental Disabilities Monitoring Network," 11 Sites, United States, 2020," *Morbidity and Mortality Weekly Report Surveillance Summaries* 2023;72(No. SS-2):1–14. http://dx.doi.org/10.15585/mmwr.ss7202a1.

We considered a host of models and proposals to help us scale up and found one investor group that valued our vision and was prepared to support what we were already doing with the resources to do more of it. Council Capital Group, a private equity firm, approached us with a congruent investment philosophy. Their involvement gave us the financial security to consider longer time horizons for the business and to expand and solidify our management structure.

We partnered with Council Capital (headquartered in Nashville, Tennessee) in 2018. Shortly after, we dramatically increased our clinical staff and brought in a new management team, including a new CEO, Kathleen Bailey Stengel, a Board Certified Behavior Analyst with concomitant business experience who shared our vision of an independent, interdisciplinary approach to neurological services.

We are not done because we know that there are many patients in need who are struggling with autism spectrum disorder and unnecessarily failing to find the services they deserve all in one place. We have helped so many people over the years who would not have reached the level they did without our help. Everyone in the communities we serve should have that opportunity.

Our quest has been renewed, and we tilt at these windmills with a stronger horse beneath us, a sharper lance, and thicker armor. We see the gaps in the system, and we remain a flexible, independent organization offering comprehensive care in ways that existing institutions and healthcare delivery systems generally cannot. We are solving problems, creating meaningful outcomes, and recently are now expanding our reach to serve patients throughout New Jersey, Pennsylvania, and other states.

And, through this book, the rest of the nation.

I will leave you with this encouraging truth as we begin our journey together toward a better way: despite the difficult times that families with neurological challenges endure, despite the emotionally taxing roller-coaster ride, despite the setbacks and apparent dead-ends, despite all of that, there is hope.

There is hope because there is a better way to treat autism spectrum disorder and other neurological issues than the methods you have encountered so far.

There is hope because scientific advances offer new diagnostic and treatment approaches, pointing us in the right direction. There is hope because these new treatment approaches have a proven track record of positive outcomes to benefit your neurodiverse loved ones.

> **This new path is an intersection of insights rather than a one-way street of prescriptions from "experts."**

There is hope because we have embraced these new approaches to forge a new path forward, and you can choose to join us on it.

On this new path, we always remember that a child is a unique human being with a family and a home life and school experiences that are part of who and what that child is. On this new path, we walk together and exchange ideas, all of us listening as well as speaking to one another. On this path, rather than confining ourselves to the pursuit of a single perspective, we incorporate all factors that may be in play.

This new path is an intersection of insights rather than a one-way street of prescriptions from "experts."

Join us on this new path as we share with you our plan for optimizing outcomes and unlocking the hopes and dreams for your child. There is hope, and now we are offering you the key.

CHAPTER 1

A Fragmented Healthcare System

D id you know? Americans spent more than $4 trillion, or nearly one-fifth of the gross domestic product (GDP), on healthcare in 2020,[3] which is three times the amount from just 2000.[4] Americans spend 50 percent more of what we earn on healthcare than residents of the country with the next most expensive healthcare system (Switzerland).[5] Nearly half of Americans say they fear a medical event could bankrupt them,[6] and for good reason. The Commonwealth Fund reports that 41 percent of working-age Americans—or seventy-

3   "Health Expenditures in the US—Statistics & Facts," Statista, August 30, 2022, https://www.statista.com/topics/6701/health-expenditures-in-the-us/#topicOverview.

4   "US National Health Expenditure as Percent of GDP from 1960 to 2021," Statista, January 9, 2023, https://www.statista.com/statistics/184968/us-health-expenditure-as-percent-of-gdp-since-1960/.

5   Irene Papanicolas et al., "Health Care Spending in the United States and Other High-Income Countries," *Journal of the American Medical Association* 319 (2018):1024–1039, doi:10.1001/jama.2018.1150.

6   Dan Winters, "50% in US Fear Bankruptcy Due to Major Health Event," Gallup, September 2020, https://news.gallup.com/poll/317948/fear-bankruptcy-due-major-health-event.aspx.

two million people—have medical bill problems or are paying off medical debt."[7]

For all that extra spending, we are rewarded with a fractured system in which care is rationed irrationally. A report in the *Journal of the American Medical Association* in 2019 found that roughly a quarter of that spending—nearly a trillion dollars—is wasted.[8] If the waste were eliminated and put back in our pockets, a family of four would get a check for $12,000 every year.

By the AMA's accounting, this waste is the result of six broad categories of inefficiency: failure of care delivery, failure of care coordination, high prices, administrative complexity, overtreatment, and low-value care.

Our patient Bobbi, who endured a tortured journey through America's healthcare system, is testament to the need for an alternative to the current delivery of care paradigm. She experienced the negative impact of all six categories of inefficiency firsthand throughout her healthcare horror story.

(Just a side note here: Bobbi is the actual name of this particular patient. We have permission to use her story and name her. When patients gave their permission to use their names, we did so. Other patients have given us permission to use their stories but not their names, so we give them aliases. Still other stories here are illustrative amalgams of real stories but not attributable to a specific person. Patient confidentiality is obviously an important aspect of our work.)

---

7   "Survey: 79 Million Americans Have Problems with Medical Bills or Debt," The Commonwealth Fund, accessed March 9, 2023, https://www.commonwealthfund. org/publications/newsletter-article/survey-79-million-americans-have-problems-medical-bills-or-debt.

8   William Shrank et al., "Waste in the US Health Care System Estimated Costs and Potential for Savings," *Journal of the American Medical Association* 322, no. 15 (2019): 1501–1509, doi: 10.1001/jama.2019.13978.

As a teenager, Bobbi suffered episodic seizures that put her in the hospital for days at a time, multiple times each month. Through a series of incorrect diagnoses, she skipped from one medication to another that seesawed her weight from a low of 90 pounds to a high of 210 pounds.

Bobbi was told she would never live a normal life, drive a car, hold a job, or have a family. A neurosurgeon proposed seizure surgery.

At that point, after a decade of hospitalizations, pharmacological experiments, endless doctors' visits, expensive diagnostic tests, and treatments, all of it had come to naught. Despite that, it had consumed hundreds of thousands of dollars, perhaps even a million or more, and it could all have been avoided.

After ten years of misery, Bobbi found our center. My astute colleague Dr. Madeline Chadehumbe listened to Bobbi's life story and ran two simple and relatively inexpensive tests: a high-density electroencephalogram (HD-EEG) and a genetic test. She determined that Bobbi had a genetic variant causing a defect in cellular calcium channels that could be treated with a low-cost medication. Her symptoms resolved nearly to the point of a cure, and she was able to resume a normal life.

For ten years, Bobbi believed that she was destined for an excruciating existence that would amount to nothing—no job, no marriage, no children—nothing to look forward to but brief reprieves between the racking seizures that gripped her body with depressing regularity.

And then, within a couple of months, thanks to two simple tests and an inexpensive medicine, Bobbi got her life back. And she has made something of it—finishing school, getting married, becoming a mother, and running her own business. She is endlessly grateful for what she views as the good fortune to finally discover the key to her condition, but viewed objectively, she could be forgiven for feeling bitterness toward a healthcare system that never took the time or engaged the right tools to find the root cause of her problems. Much to her credit, Bobbi chooses to focus on the positive aspect of the end of her suffering, but we have to ask: Why did she have to suffer—for ten years, no less—in the first place?

THE DIAGNOSTIC ODYSSEY

The primary difference between Bobbi's story and the thousands out there involving diagnostic odysseys without answers or solutions is that Bobbi's has a happy ending. Bobbi's is just one story among thousands of patients daily who present with a set of symptoms viewed by specialists through a single lens. Their intervention strategy devours time, energy, and significant financial resources chasing predetermined treatments uninhibited by contrary scientific evidence. Often, patients make repeated emergency room visits and require inpatient hospital stays at a daily cost of thousands of dollars. Aside from the pain and suffering endured by patients and their families, the process is stunningly inefficient and expensive. The pari-mutuel nature of healthcare financing ensures that the ballooning costs from these kinds of situations find their way into your insurance premiums—and everyone else's.

The quixotic search for a functional diagnosis of illnesses and conditions is so common that "diagnostic odyssey" is a recognized term in medical literature. A global commission was formed in 2018 to end diagnostic odysseys for children with rare diseases, in recognition of the fact that "the consequences can be devastating: delays in treatment that could save a child's life or, when there is no treatment or cure, robbing families of peace of mind and the ability to plan for their child's future."[9] The Child Neurology Foundation established an

---

9   Simon Kos et al., "Letter from the Co-chairs," Global Rare Disease Commission, accessed March 9, 2023, https://www.globalrarediseasecommission.com/co-chairs.

education initiative in 2020 that focused on shortening the diagnostic odyssey, as there may be as many as four hundred million people worldwide who suffer from diseases that take an average of five years to diagnose. A French study underway as we write this is studying assessments capable of shortening the diagnostic odysseys of patients with severe neurodevelopmental disorders.

In short, more people around the world suffer from undiagnosed conditions than the entire populations of the United States and Canada. That doesn't stop clinicians from offering barely supported guesses, prescribing poorly tolerated medications in a kind of hunt-and-peck experiment, and even, in Bobbi's case, proposing brain surgery.

From the first descriptions of autism, the diagnostic odyssey took thirty years, not to name the condition but to pinpoint the source. In the absence of evidence, in trying to identify a common source of the condition, medical professionals blamed poor mothering. They coined the term "refrigerator mothers" to describe those who were cold, neglectful, and even abusive.

They came to this conclusion by watching autistic children, who almost uniformly failed to bond with their mothers. The children ignored their mothers and showed no affection toward them. Consequently, the medical profession concluded that parenting must be the issue. Psychiatrist Leo Kanner, who was most responsible for the refrigerator mother theory, said of the children, "They were kept neatly in refrigerators, which did not defrost."

Psychologist Bruno Bettleheim, a concentration camp survivor, published a book in 1967 called *The Empty Fortress*, comparing the demeanor of autistic children's parents to Nazi guards at concentration camps.[10] The effect on parents, already suffering, already des-

---

10   Bruno Bettleheim, *The Empty Fortress: Infantile Autism and the Birth of the Self* (New York City: Free Press, 1972).

perately attempting to break through to uncommunicative children lost in unseen worlds, was devastating. Varnished with a patina of science, this profound insult was a generally accepted attack on the very essence of mothers and fathers across the country.

Perhaps worse, it set back efforts to diagnose and treat autism because it diverted attention to the perceived failures of parents and turned a biological issue into a subject of familial shame. Who knows how many parents, fearful of the stigma, attempted to hide their children's condition rather than treat it?

We see this ourselves in the twenty-first century. We often work with guilt-ridden parents, such as one family whose son was so severely autistic that he needed to be institutionalized. They came to us for a full diagnostic workup, and we found a molecular mutation in his genes associated with autism. When we revealed this to his mother, she began to cry, not because finding the source of her son's condition was going to lead to any treatment breakthroughs but because she could, for the first time as his mother, assign the fault to something besides herself. She told us she had always believed she must have done something wrong. Bettleheim would have approved of that notion, but of course, it was a dangerous misconception.

By the 1970s, the refrigerator mother theory had largely been debunked, although the exact cause or causes of autism are still not well understood. It is widely accepted today that genetics play an oversized role, but external factors and acquired insults, sometimes in conjunction with an underlying genetic predisposition, have also impacted the rising incidences of autism. The rate of children with autism spectrum disorders has tripled between 2000 and 2020, in part due to better diagnostics and in part due to unexplained factors. We know for sure that there is no association between autism and the quality of parenting.[11]

Because autism may have multiple catalysts and affects social, emotional, psychological, cognitive, and physical functions, there is no one way to treat an autistic child. Moreover, as autism affects a child's whole life, and the life of his or her entire family, many congruent interventions are necessary. Thus, we believe it is imperative for medical professionals to take a holistic and interdisciplinary approach to caring for each child, which is not a normative process in the current healthcare environment.

> **We believe it is imperative for medical professionals to take a holistic and interdisciplinary approach to caring for each child, which is not a normative process in the current healthcare environment.**

A FRAGMENTED HEALTHCARE SYSTEM

Case in point: Eleven-year-old Charlie (not his real name) came to us with a diagnosis of Asperger syndrome, a disorder on the autism spectrum with symptoms that appear less severe than autism (Asperger syndrome has been eliminated as an official diagnosis in recent years, although it is still used by some to describe certain individuals with high-functioning autism). Charlie stared off into space and made self-injurious threats. As you can imagine, this caused his mother high anxiety.

---

11   Mark Mintz, "Evolution in the Understanding of Autism Spectrum Disorder: Historical Perspective," *The Indian Journal of Pediatrics* 84 (2017): 44–52, doi: 10.1007/s12098-016-2080-8.

We listened intently to his mother's narrative and then observed him repeatedly in myriad situations. We engaged a multidisciplinary approach, incorporating multiple perspectives and a range of expertise. Charlie was evaluated by our neuropsychology team, directed by Dr. Gregory Alberts, who specializes in clinical neuropsychology and has wide-ranging experience and expertise in the assessment and treatment of individuals with acquired or developmentally based neurological impairment.

Next, Charlie worked on his social skills with our behavioral therapists, led by Dr. Kaori Nepo, an internationally respected, board-certified behavior analyst (BCBA) who has done extensive research on the use of commonly available technology for behavior interventions. (BCBA certification is designated by the Behavior Analyst Certification Board, Inc.®) Our pediatric neurologist, Dr. Ronald Barabas, a physician skilled in evaluating and treating brain disorders and diseases, ordered an advanced technology high-definition electroencephalography (HD-EEG) study of Charlie's brain, and our medical geneticist, Dr. Richard Boles, who specializes in finding abnormalities at the molecular level, reanalyzed Charlie's entire genetic sequence to assess for a genetic issue.

It took a team of clinicians working collaboratively to diagnose Charlie's various physical, social, psychological, and emotional disabilities and develop a successful treatment plan moving forward. This was facilitated by an organization like ours with an integrated, multidisciplinary assessment and treatment paradigm. Typically, this kind of comprehensive diagnostic workup would be fragmented and difficult to accomplish, even within a single institution. Our practice eliminates multiple referrals and separate visits to various independent specialists and guarantees robust communication among the various professionals involved. Payers and healthcare policy makers have paid scant attention over the years to "the robust interdisciplinary communication necessary for comprehensive care," but it is integral to our practice because it is critical to good outcomes.[12]

We found two complications beyond Asperger syndrome that were interfering with Charlie's progress. One was a subclinical series of abnormal electrical discharges in his brain without overt behavioral changes that a clinical seizure would produce. The ability to detect these occult electrical discharges was made possible by HD-EEG and may have been missed with previous conventional EEG. The other was a processing issue that prevented Charlie from mental organization, and problem-solving ("executive functioning"), and "working memory" (if you think of your brain as a computer, Charlie's RAM was failing to store data needed to piece together puzzles of information). Correctly tracing the biological and clinical sources of his issues was step one in drawing the blueprint for successful treatment.

Previous research, including from our own group,[13] has suggested that suppressing subclinical electrical discharges of the brain with certain medications can lead to improvement in working memory, language, and behavior. Because Charlie had a lot on his plate, considering the academic and social challenges of school, ABA therapy, and the problem-solving issues, it was important that we prescribed a medication for the electrical discharges without serious side effects. We utilized one that suppressed these tiny neurological lightning bolts while we provided behavioral aids that helped with his verbal and

12   Maria Theodorou, Bruce Henschen, and Margaret Chapman, "The Comprehensive Care Plan: A Patient-Centered, Multidisciplinary Communication Tool for Frequently Hospitalized Patients," *Journal of Quality Patient Satisfaction* 46, no. 4 (April 2020): 217–226, doi: 10.1016/j.jcjq.2020.01.002.

13   Mark Mintz et al., "The Under-Recognized Epilepsy Spectrum: The Effects of Levetiracetam on Neuropsychological Functioning in Relation to Subclinical Spike Production," *Journal of Child Neurology* 24, no. 7 (July 2009): 807–815, doi: 10.1177/0883073808330762.

social interactions and helped him learn and organize, with overall improvements in cognitive functioning, academic productivity, and verbal and nonverbal social communication.

Four years later, Charlie is off the medicine, and his HD-EEGs have normalized. Academically, he is an average high school student receiving cognitive behavioral therapy so that he can establish his own social strategies and compensating behaviors. The individual education program (IEP) that we helped his school develop for him goes well beyond narrow in-class observations to include all the therapies he needs for a rich home, school, and community life. Hardly a social butterfly, Charlie is learning strategies to make friends and join peer groups. If you saw him on the school campus, he would blend in with the sea of teenage interactions and idiosyncrasies observable at any secondary school.

SILOED TREATMENT: THE BLIND MEN AND THE ELEPHANT

Autism spectrum disorders primarily affect the nervous system, but there are numerous associated health issues and significant impacts on family structures. Programs lacking coordinated assessment and treatment across medical and behavioral services hearken to the proverbial blind men and the elephant, each exploring a different body part and universalizing their narrow conclusions.

In the parable, a group of blind men encounter a single elephant but draw different conclusions about their experience. One man touches the elephant's leg and conceptualizes the unknown beast as a tree. Another man touches the elephant's trunk and believes he has grasped a snake. The third man, who touches the tusk, is convinced that the elephant is a spear, the man at its side, a wall, and so on. The analogous siloed treatment of patients with multisystem involvement like Charlie is patently suboptimal, yet that regimen remains the rule rather than the exception.

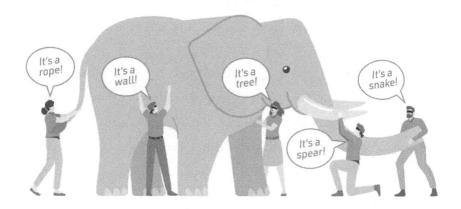

I noticed this as early as my pediatric residency at Albert Einstein College of Medicine/Montefiore Medical Center in the Bronx, New York, during the early days of the AIDS epidemic. Children were presenting at Einstein in the mid-'80s with strange, opportunistic infections like *pneumocystis pneumonia* and cytomegalovirus, and clinicians were flummoxed. No one was connecting the dots between the AIDS epidemic and pediatric disorders because children were not transmitting bodily fluids through unprotected sex or intravenous drug use (the common means of transmitting HIV infection in adults).

Except, of course, they were. HIV, the virus that causes AIDS, was being passed through the umbilical cord by infected mothers to their fetuses. Alternatively, some infants and children became infected from tainted blood transfusions. In both cases, babies were exposed to HIV without engaging in any high-risk behavior.

It took a while for healthcare professionals to make the connection and realize that newborn babies were entering the world with HIV infections. Until that point, there was a dearth of attention paid to the HIV status of pregnant women and no conversation with HIV-positive women about the dangers inherent to mother and child of becoming pregnant. We had not yet connected the dots.

In 1986, I began a fellowship in child neurology at the New Jersey Medical School in Newark, New Jersey. As part of a multidisciplinary pediatric AIDS center, I began to see how breaking down silos among practitioners accelerated the diagnosis of underlying conditions and generated comprehensive and innovative treatments. The clinicians there recognized then that HIV affects many different organ systems as well as family dynamics and psychosocial functioning. In that program, specialists in infectious disease, pulmonology, immunology, neurology, social work, nursing, and many other areas of expertise shared an urgency to determine optimal treatments by combining their myriad insights in a synergistic way.

Other professionals at NeurAbilities share similar stories. The therapists who work with us encountered the same gaps from the behavioral perspective. They tell us how they witnessed behavioral specialists—therapists employing empirically proven ABA therapies in the treatment of autistic children—being sidelined by the medical community as not being a valued component of the treatment process. In response, therapists developed their own siloed practices and their own resistance to medical input.

Here is one story our CEO, Kathleen Bailey Stengel, tells us repeatedly about the inadequacy of a fragmented system vividly displayed during her early training. It involves the treatment of a three-year-old girl diagnosed by the medical community with autism and referred for early intervention services.

Upon initial intake, the early intervention team noted significant hand-mouthing that was causing damage to the skin. The little girl was constantly sucking on her hand and parts of her forearm, causing rashes and bleeding. The treating pediatrician did little to coordinate care with the team, regardless of the data provided by the therapists. It was even suggested that she would "grow out of it."

The behavior team continued to analyze data taken during treatment with no clear pattern to make a useful behavioral intervention. The team continued to provide data to the physician team with little interaction or acknowledgment for close to six months. Upon the child's first visit to a dentist, it was discovered that, in fact, the child had a tooth abscess, and she lacked the skills to communicate it.

Her issue was not psychological or behavioral but was physical and social. Because she was labeled "autistic," her behavior was being viewed exclusively through a narrow lens, with the result that this three-year-old was made to suffer for half a year with an easily resolved medical issue. That is why we constantly remind ourselves that we are diagnosis agnostic. We tailor our treatment to the needs of the patient without regard for the name of the disorder attached to them. Unfortunately, such a clinical model is relatively rare.

THE MULTIDISCIPLINARY IMPERATIVE

Consider a thought experiment about the value of neurologists. Manifestly, they are critical healthcare practitioners. These physicians who study the brain and nervous system, which affect literally every aspect of our physical, cognitive, and emotional lives, are essential to maintaining health among our citizens. Neurologists are highly educated experts who spend their entire twenties learning their profession before they can work unsupervised. They complete the rigors of medical school, followed by four years of hands-on residency training under the guidance of other physicians (five years for pediatric neurologists). Many neurologists add another year or two of subspecialty fellowship on top of that, focusing their neurology specialty on, for example, epilepsy. In all, they spend about a decade gaining the skills and expertise to diagnose and treat patients with a host of neurological disorders like autism.

Neuropsychologists/psychologists, the clinicians who study the mind and its effects on conscious and unconscious behavior, travel a different path to their "doctor" status. It also includes years of study and specialized training. The indispensable role neuropsychologists/psychologists play in diagnosing and treating the one in five Americans suffering with mental illncss is also plainly evident. Although the clinical practice of psychology, like medicine, is a mixture of art and science, it would be hard to imagine a functional healthcare system without psychologists.

Finally, consider behavior therapists. The therapy with the most empirical research proving measurable positive outcomes in patients with autism spectrum disorders is applied behavior analysis (ABA), as practiced by behavioral therapists. ABA therapy interventions produce socialization among neurodiverse children in a neurotypical society every day. The value of these experts is also evident, as they do hands-on work with a rapidly growing portfolio of ASD patients to help them become functioning, independent adults capable of reaching their full potential.

In our organization alone, we employ all those named above in addition to the expertise of medical geneticists, developmental-behavioral pediatricians, advanced practice nurses, creative arts therapists, and more. Each brings a unique perspective and knowledge base to the cases of children and their families who seek our services. Beyond that, we communicate with a host of other experts in fields outside our areas of knowledge. It is imperative to do so. Lacking that variety limits the understanding of patients' issues.

The theoretical underpinnings of each field of study are its own, leaving experts in different fields with different perspectives, much the way different national cultures imbue people with different perspectives. The construct within which psychologists approach a patient problem is different from that within which a neurologist works. One is focused on the physical structures of the brain and nervous system while the other is more concerned with the mind, a nonphysical manifestation of the brain. The two approach cases differently; consequently, they may reach different conclusions after observing the same patient.

Any individual clinician with a specific focus and perspective is constrained by the paradigm in which he or she operates. A plethora of practitioners grounded in their various unique practice models brings a diversity of perspectives more likely to unlock the most vexing clinical issues. Our independent, multidisciplinary practice is designed to deliver just these results.

Indeed, if "follow the money" is the mantra explaining everything from politics to healthcare, it is easy to see why the independent, multidisciplinary approach is not the norm. Funding sources actively hinder this approach by reimbursing each individual element of the process separately and offering nothing for applying an integrated approach. In fact, there are regulatory barriers to such an approach: in most instances, behavior therapists engage in wild goose chases just to read the neurologist's report.

> Indeed, if "follow the money" is the mantra explaining everything from politics to healthcare, it is easy to see why the independent, multidisciplinary approach is not the norm.

(In our practice, information is shared among the treating clinicians.) Insurers and government funders allow reimbursement for medical intervention in one box, behavioral intervention in another, and so on, with different, often contradictory regulations for each. Any enterprise inclined to establish a multidisciplinary approach would have to be seriously motivated to do so because the system inherently discourages this model.

OVERCOMING YEARS OF TRAINING

Understandably, healthcare providers often approach diagnostics and therapeutics through a narrow lens of their discipline, which fosters a natural orientation to practice in silos. Yet we are complex organisms dependent on the interplay and coordination of various organ systems' biological processes, and likewise, optimal care and management of complicated disorders like autism require healthcare professionals to interface and collaborate with those in other clinical and scientific fields of expertise. This sounds like common sense, but the present structure and incentives of our healthcare system create many obstacles to achieving a multidisciplinary approach to healthcare. This dilemma is magnified in treating those with neurodevelopmental disabilities and neurobehavioral disorders.

Take any example you want from virtually any other industry, and consider how quickly a company would fail if it isolated its thought leaders from each other. How long could an automobile company persist if the engine designers failed to take into account the space requirements under the hood or in the passenger compartment, or emissions issues, or gas mileage requirements? Imagine them not just failing to integrate their innovations with the other departments in the company but being actively discouraged from doing so by corporate brass. This company would fail spectacularly in the marketplace. Yet that is the paradigm in healthcare.

This issue reverberates in our practice on many levels, despite our total dedication to a multidisciplinary team approach. To assemble such a team starts with identifying professionals and support staff who not only share our core values but also a willingness and motivation to learn and function within an innovative healthcare delivery model that is different from the mainstream. Rather than the usual recruitment approach of filling open positions, we attempt to identify talented professionals and create positions that will utilize their skills and abilities for the patients we serve. In the disciplines serving special needs populations, there is a shortage of clinical specialists. Yet the distinctiveness and independence of our organization have attracted open-minded experts who have made a difference in the lives of those we serve.

We hire unique and talented people whose extraordinary skills encompass areas not generally valued by other institutions. We seek those with a humanistic ethos most squarely in line with ours. They must be open-minded enough to recognize that the perspectives and orientations of other practitioners might be superior in a given situation.

We knew a behavior analyst with incomparable skills and the mindset of a musician in an orchestra whose primary concern is complementing the other instruments. Her experience was primarily focused on adolescents, as opposed to our need for behavior analysts to provide early intervention by age three. Nonetheless, we hired her, to our mutual delight, and she has risen to a management position, evangelizing our values to other staff and potential partners. Had we been hiring based solely on résumés, we might have missed this diamond.

Having said that, all our clinicians do have outstanding professional credentials. It turns out that some of the highest achievers in our fields have reached our conclusions independently.

THE OVERUSE OF MEDICATION

The default position in modern medical care is less to understand the cause of symptoms than to suppress them, usually with medication. In this healthcare model, if the medication fails, the alternative is more or different medication until all medication options are exhausted. Only then is the full spectrum of causes of disease considered. This is not confined to general medical care but also is prevalent in diseases of the brain that are hard to pinpoint the way, for example, an allergy, broken leg, or strep throat may be. It is easier to fall back on pharmacology than to engage in the detective work required for a full understanding of the problem and offer a road map to effective treatment.

Case in point: A nonverbal eight-year-old boy was referred to our office following several years of ineffective treatment. In fact, Aidan's (not his real name) quality of life had been degrading during the time he was being treated by his pediatrician and a psychologist, placed in special classes, and offered behavioral support in school.

In other words, two doctors' offices and a dozen or more educators and administrators provided their professional expertise and caring hearts to Aidan, yet his condition worsened, placing ever more stress on his family. Aidan was experiencing continuous pain and inflicting wanton destruction in his wake. He was aggressive in his behavior to those around him and prone to occasional, unexplained violence. His meltdowns put himself, other people, and property in danger and caused immense anxiety at home and at school.

In American healthcare today, the reflexive corrective for this type of behavior is to find the magic chemical that will subdue Aidan's behavior. He arrived in our offices on a cocktail of medications that included Adderall, a psychostimulant; risperidone, an antipsychotic; and clonazepam, a sedative that can reduce anxiety but also suppress seizures. These pharmaceuticals will be familiar to many parents of autistic children. They are designed for the symptoms that Aidan was displaying.

There are two problems with this formula. First, medications have unintended consequences. The side effects of the drug combination were insomnia and a 20 percent weight gain that pushed Aidan into the obesity category. Even if this pharmacological regimen had ameliorated his symptoms, it would have come with a substantial cost. Second, a child is not a collection of symptoms; he is a unique human propelled to act by his biology and psychology. Simply prescribing medication is easy, but it fails to address underlying biological and clinical causes and contributions. This was the case for Aidan, whose symptoms got no better and whose overall health declined.

In our office, we have adopted a philosophy of using the minimal effective dose of medicine possible. "Start low; go slow" is our mantra. If we can treat a child without introducing chemicals into their body, that is optimal. To the extent that pharmaceuticals are necessary, the less, the better, for exactly the reason that drugs have side effects and alter the body's natural chemistry. Before we prescribe medicine, we fully investigate the cause of symptoms in the

> In our office, we have adopted a philosophy of using the minimal effective dose of medicine possible. "Start low; go slow" is our mantra.

hope that we might find the underlying problem, which can lead us to discover an alternative way to address it.

In our initial evaluation of Aidan, we were determined to understand why his behaviors were occurring and whether something biological or psychological was setting them off. We simultaneously weaned him off drugs that were demonstrating no clear efficacy. Our behavioral team conducted a functional behavior analysis in his natural setting—not in our office, as many therapists do, but in Aidan's home. Our behavior analysts discovered that Aidan's outbursts were attention-seeking strategies that worked splendidly. School personnel and his parents had been trained to respond to them with reprimands and corrective action, thus inadvertently fueling further negative behaviors. Instead, our behavior analysts initiated parent training to recognize these behavior patterns and institute reactions that included ignoring and redirecting. Immediately, the outbursts subsided.

While Aidan ceased to be a physical threat to himself and those around him, he nonetheless remained prone to occasional escalations, verbal outbursts, hyperactivity, and agitation. Doing a bit of detective work, one of our neurologists homed in on a pattern and determined that Aidan experienced "autonomic over-responsivity"—that is, poor regulation of physiological responses to environmental stimulation. Additional testing with HD-EEG found an additional biological issue in his brain that caused an unregulated response to his environment. We removed him from all his other meds and put him on one low-dose medication without serious side effects, which has calmed the flare-ups.

Aidan is not cured by any means, but we have alleviated the severe behaviors and made his situation manageable for him, his family, and his school. Both Aidan and his family can now enjoy a more normal life without fear of violence and destruction. The behavioral supports he continues to receive are helping him navigate the world around him. All that was necessary to reach this more optimal state was to replace the drugs-first mentality with an effort to determine the source of his behavior and use medicine only when necessary for his specific case.

Aidan's story stands as yet another in a parade of data points demonstrating how medical science often falls back on the medication shortcut. Pharmacology can be an efficacious adjunct to other forms of treatment, but it must be based on a thorough understanding of a condition's biological source.

Consider this lament by the American Psychological Association in 2010 about the trend toward pharmaceuticals and away from psychotherapy to treat mental health issues. It quoted a government survey that found more than 57 percent of patients were being treated with medication only, a dramatic spike from just a few years earlier.

Psychotherapy doesn't need a "black-box" warning. It doesn't cause common side effects, such as weight gain, nausea, sexual dysfunction, or sleep disturbance. It doesn't stop working altogether when treatment ends. In fact, psychotherapy arms users with a new set of problem-solving skills they can apply whenever needed.[14]

The APA editorial blamed Big Pharma's relentless advertising, which has only intensified in the intervening years, and topped $5 billion in 2016, by many accounts. That figure is for all drugs (not just psychotropics) and for all patients (not just children), but the trends are the same across the board, as the APA's editorial suggests. It appears that clinicians have been complicit in Big Pharma's induced supply-side market pressures to create the impetus for the vast overprescription of pharmaceuticals.

If this sounds familiar, you may be remembering the opioid crisis, which burst onto the headlines in 2016 when forty-two thousand Americans died from the abuse of commonly prescribed narcotics.[15] Physicians were encouraged to prescribe these substances by pharmaceutical companies, which soft-pedaled the risk of addiction and abuse. Pills are easy to prescribe, covered by insurance, and sold by companies that curry favor with physicians in a variety of ways.

---

14   Katherine Nordal, "Where Has All the Psychotherapy Gone?," *American Psychological Association: Perspectives on Practice* 41, no. 10 (2010): 17, https://www.apa.org/monitor/2010/11/perspectives.

15   US Government Accountability Office, "Opioid Crisis: Status of Public Health Emergency Authorities," GAO-18-685R, September 26, 2018, https://www.gao.gov/products/gao-18-685r.

A 2018 study in *JAMA Internal Medicine* found a correlation between the number of prescriptions for opioids written by physicians and the number of meals or incentive payments they received from the drugmaker. From this and other information, there has been subsequent tightening of regulations concerning the interactions between Big Pharma and physicians.[16]

The poster child for this is Purdue Pharma, makers of hydromorphone, oxycodone, fentanyl, codeine, and hydrocodone. Their signature pain medication, OxyContin, which earned the company $2.8 billion between 1995 and 2001, was marketed to physicians with the promise that it provided "smooth and sustained pain control all day and all night" while exposing patients to less potential for abuse because of its time-release properties.[17] There was no scientific evidence for this; indeed, the US Justice Department determined the company was aware that pills were being crushed and snorted, stolen from pharmacies, and sold for high value on the street—all signs that they were being abused. The company supplemented its marketing by wooing physicians aggressively with junkets, paid speaking engagements, and other enticements. The company had created a web of supporters and enablers in the medical community.

Eventually, as the deaths piled up and the nation recognized a crisis situation, dozens of states sued Purdue Pharma for billions of dollars. The Sackler family, which owned and controlled the company,

16   Scott Hadland et al., "Association of Pharmaceutical Industry Marketing of Opioid Products to Physicians with Subsequent Opioid Prescribing," JAMA Internal Medicine 178, no. 6 (2018): 861–863 , doi: 10.1001/jamainternmed.2018.1999.

17   Harriet Ryan, Lisa Girion and Scott Glover, "'You Want a Description of Hell?' OxyContin's 12-Hour Problem", *LA Times*, May 5, 2016, https://www.latimes.com/projects/oxycontin-part1/.

settled the case for $8 billion, including more than $3.5 billion in criminal penalties, and relinquished control of the company.[18]

Left in the wake of this tragedy are millions of ordinary people left addicted to pain medications and a cascade of health issues that could have been easily prevented. Many of them could have been treated in other ways rather than a pill.

TRAIN-THE-PARENT MYTH IN AUTISM

One model of early intervention for autism involves training the parent to provide ABA therapy around the clock rather than for a limited prescribed number of hours per week, as a therapist might do. The theory behind this is similar to the notion that it would be more effective to train a business owner to maintain their own accounting ledger rather than hire a bookkeeper. Although parent training and intervention is a useful complement, replacing ABA therapy with parent-led therapy is suboptimal.

The more apt comparison would be to train a parent to do their own orthodontic work on a child who needs braces or to learn the basics of law so they can represent themselves in legal proceedings. ABA therapists are educated professionals, usually with master's degree preparation, certification in the science of applied behavior analysis, and expertise in autism spectrum disorders. ABA therapists spend years practicing and honing their craft. What they do is not something that can be summarized in an hour and turned over to the responsibility of parents. That is unfair to parents and children alike.

In some states, parents are required to attend ABA training to qualify for services. This creates an unnecessary barrier to care for

---

18   Corey Davis, "The Purdue Pharma Opioid Settlement: Accountability, or Just the Cost of Doing Business?" *New England Journal of Medicine* 384 (2021): 97–99, doi: 10.1056/NEJMp2033382.

those who need it most. That is not to say that providing parents with additional skills is unhelpful; indeed, it is an ordinary expectation of a therapist's work. Parent training is written into school IEPs, not as a substitute for therapy but as a complement to intensive professional behavior analysis. Numerous courses for parents exist both online and in person that teach practical strategies, providing parents a framework for understanding their children's conditions and ameliorating their social, communication, and behavioral issues.

In short, we heartily endorse training parents as an extension of therapy. But if training parents becomes a replacement for therapy, it is a recipe for failure—at the expense of the children and everyone around them.

To be clear, our multidisciplinary arrangement is no panacea. There is a certain efficiency in a solitary voice, in a consensus of ideas. Our integrated approach presents many challenges beyond the strangling bureaucracy of the healthcare system. Requesting multiple opinions from different perspectives means receiving multiple opinions from different perspectives—each convinced that they are right. Because the professionals in each discipline are trained to take a unique approach, each problem we confront is answered from multiple unique approaches, not always harmoniously. Researchers, scientists, and clinicians view problems in different ways that are often synergistic but sometimes contradictory, even mutually exclusive. Our teams have many robust discussions about how best to treat our patients and optimize outcomes, not just at the tactical or even strategic level but also right down to the fundamentals of what it means to be a human. It is intellectually invigorating—and also challenging.

As I say, it is a challenge, ultimately one we believe—we know—is worth the struggle. Working together is harder than working alone, but our patients benefit from the diversity of ideas and philosophies we bring to bear on each patient's situation. We consider the extra time we take a short-term investment in a long-term optimized outcome, very much akin to the way setting aside part of our income into a retirement fund serves our retirement needs years later. In fact, cast in that light, the payoff is much more immediate. The small sacrifices required to collaborate pay immense dividends in days, weeks, or months for our patients.

Evidently, we're not alone in that calculation. The American Academy of Neurology has awarded us the seminal 2023 Neurology Practice Award in recognition of our innovative solutions that improve the practice of neurology and patient care. Our "one-stop-shop" clinical model, quality outcomes, and community outreach and service activities particularly impressed the judges. In 2008, we were also given a New Jersey Autism Clinical Centers-Clinical Enhancement Grant from the Governor's Council for Medical Research and Treatment of Autism.

Our integrated clinical model has included clinical research, giving patients access to new or experimental treatments available only through clinical research trials. Additionally, our staff have been awarded funding for investigator-initiated grants testing and exploring various scientific hypotheses. This has resulted in the ongoing academic productivity of our clinicians through presentations and lectures at major national and international scientific meetings and conferences, publications throughout medical and scientific literature, and providing training to undergraduate and postgraduate clinicians and trainees. Thus, we have been able to demonstrate the ability to replicate an academic and research environment integrated with a clinical service model—but in an independent organization.

THE DILEMMA OF GUARANTEEING MEASURABLE OUTCOMES

On a given day at our center, a mother and her child with ASD walk in, and the mother makes a very reasonable proposal: "Guarantee that you will achieve some tangible outcome with my child, and I will hire you."

We hear some form of this offer regularly. No one wants to invest the time, effort, and expense on the hope that something good might come of it—but might not.

As I say, it is not an unreasonable expectation. When you take your car to the shop for a brake job, you want the brakes working when you drive it home. Anything less would be unsatisfactory, and you would likely return to the service station expecting them to correct the issue for free. If your child broke a leg, you would expect the orthopedist to set it correctly and for healing to commence at the standard pace.

> **Brains are not bones or brakes; they are mysterious and somewhat inaccessible organs, each one unique to its user and buffeted by inputs from the internal and external life of the owner.**

Anything less would be considered a failure.

We have over fifteen years of experience producing extraordinary results for our patients, many of whom came to us as a last resort after years of suffering along their diagnostic and therapeutic odyssey. But brains are not bones or brakes; they are mysterious and somewhat inaccessible organs, each one unique to its user and buffeted by inputs from the internal and external life of the owner. There is simply no way to guarantee a particular outcome to any parent, child, or family.

We do offer a different path, one that is logically superior to the conventional methods and is supported by empirical evidence. It starts with our multidisciplinary/interdisciplinary/transdisciplinary approach, which benefits from the synergistic involvement of the myriad services and expertise a patient with neurological issues might require. It is supported by our holistic view of each patient, recognizing that their experiences extend far beyond our exam room and affect family members and others besides just themselves. It continues with our clinical model, which seeks to understand and identify biological causes and contributions to disorders and diseases. It culminates in being able to provide "personalized" and "precision" treatment strategies and regimens. Patients who employ our unique services benefit from an independent agency unfettered from an institutional bureaucracy, which is, therefore, nimble and innovative in ways that a larger enterprise cannot be. No wonder our organization has grown many times over during the past decade.

That is not to say that we do not have tangible evidence of the value of our coordinated approach to neurological issues. We track outcomes in our office and can report many positive results.

Our patients experience many fewer hospital visits than patients being treated through traditional methods. Patients required two or more hospital visits annually much more often when their conditions were being managed by previous providers compared to when they were being managed by us. How much more? Two-and-a-half times as much. Even if a parent's only goal for their child is to prevent endless hospitalizations, enlisting our services would be beneficial.

In 2016, the American Academy of Neurology and Child Neurology Society established a set of standard quality measures for child neurology practice. Among these recommendations are genetic testing for neuro-developmental disorders and services for transitioning from pediatric neurology to adult neurology.[19] Our practice routinely subscribes to nine of the eleven recommendations (with the remaining two not relevant to our patient population); in fact, the large majority of our patients receive genetic testing, and we have fully resolved the issue of transitioning adolescent patients to adult services by offering life-span services.

Of course, that is not the only value of the care we provide.

In previous surveys, two-thirds of our patients reported overall improvement in the coordination of their care with us, and as a result, a majority reported improvement in behavior, academic performance, and a host of other outcomes. The baseline for this comparison is not a standing start in most cases: these are often patients who were seen by other practitioners prior to their involvement with us.

The experience of visiting our offices shapes the way patients and their parents feel about our service. From the moment patients walk in the door, they should be greeted warmly. Staff should treat them with respect, listen carefully to their concerns, and educate them about the treatment every step of the way. Our patients express overwhelming satisfaction with those elements of their visits, offering written comments about our doctors and support staff filled with terms like "tremendous," "outstanding," "impressive," and "absolutely wonderful." Patients and their families have expressed frequently that they felt the doctor listened to their concerns, and a large majority would recommend us to a friend.

For most children with neurological disorders, our goal is to help them become independent, functioning adults. Families we work with know that we are their committed partners working toward that goal. Research shows that for 10 to 20 percent of children with autism

---

19   "Child Neurology: Quality Measurement Set," American Academy of Neurology Institute, December 2016, https://www. https://www.aan.com/siteassets/ home-page/policy-and-guidelines/quality/quality-measures/child-neurology/16child neurologymeasures_pg.pdf.

under the age of five, intensive treatment can help them resolve their issues to the point that they shed the diagnosis.[20] That does not suggest a "cure," just that they can "recover" and be indistinguishable from their peers. They are the lucky ones.

Other children's brains are different. They may be further along the autism spectrum with other confounding disabilities. For them, an optimized outcome may be something less than independence but nonetheless a more productive and fulfilling life than they currently experience. That may not sound like a satisfactory alternative to you, but it might mean the world to that child and their family.

> **Our guarantee is that we will never stop trying and will never forget that a child with a neurological disorder has a family who also suffers.**

The point is, there is no secret sauce or magic formula for children with autism spectrum disorder or other neurological impairments, nor can anyone credibly promise some specific level of success. Our guarantee is that we will never stop trying and will never forget that a child with a neurological disorder has a family who also suffers.

This is what we tell the parents who come to us seeking guarantees. We're honest about not being able to promise any particular outcome. We guarantee that if a positive outcome is feasible, we will do everything we possibly can to achieve it. Most people appreciate our honesty, accept our empirical support, and agree to become patients.

We never stop trying, even for those whose stories we know will not have happy endings.

---

20   Deborah Anderson et al., "Predicting Young Adult Outcome among More and Less Cognitively Able Individuals with Autism Spectrum Disorders," *Journal of Psychiatry and Psychology* 55, no. 5 (2014): 485–494, doi: 10.1111/jcpp.12178.

I'll share one family's sad journey, which we have joined. We believe the family would testify that our team has been a welcome and indispensable partner along the way.

Amanda (not her real name) is going to die, not sometime in the future like most of us, but soon. She has an incurable degenerative disease caused by an inherited enzyme deficiency that manifests itself in increasing behavioral disturbances and brain degeneration culminating in death. Now over twenty-one, Amanda has already exceeded her life expectancy and is living on borrowed time.

Given this diagnosis, Amanda's doctors were at a loss to help her and told the family simply and repeatedly that she was going to die. Her behavior deteriorated to the point where she was no longer verbal, no longer able to ambulate on her own, and no longer in control of her bodily functions. She experienced episodic headaches that increased the severity of her behavioral outbursts.

Amanda's parents care for her, and they are resigned to her fate. But in the meantime, they want her to have an optimal quality of life. When they came to us, we offered no promises except that we would do everything we could to help her. We found the source of her headaches and administered medicine that resolved them. We continue to battle alongside the family to ameliorate any pain she might experience and to ease the most severe behavioral flare-ups. We have not cured Amanda, nor are we able to do much to extend her life. For her family, an optimized outcome is to have a team of dedicated medical professionals acknowledging their emotional pain and their daughter's suffering, accompanying them on their journey, and working relentlessly to soften Amanda's eventual landing.

Ultimately, that is our guarantee: we never give up on our patients, no matter how intractable the problems, no matter the obstacles. We offer children, adolescents, and adults realistic hope that they can have a better quality of life, whatever that might mean for them. We stand beside families thrust into lives infused with neurological issues and offer the promise to be their partners and exhaust every resource to achieve whatever we and they together describe as "success" for their child. We are a team of many passionate professionals who entered our professions to provide hope to children and families, and that is what we do every single day.

The conventional healthcare system has other priorities than producing optimized outcomes of patients with pediatric neurological and neurodevelopmental disorders like autism. The focus is on individual, siloed care—disconnected from the expertise of related disciplines, disruptive of beneficial interdisciplinary communication, shackled to a bureaucratic institution with multiple conflicting priorities, producing diagnoses and treatment decisions narrowed by blinders and often contrary to the interest of patients. There is no reimbursement system for caring about families and the impact of a child's condition on parents, siblings, and others. Nor is there any recognition that pediatric patients—or any patients for that matter—are whole beings who have home lives, school lives, work lives, and so on, each of which must be considered when planning treatment.

> Ultimately, that is our guarantee: we never give up on our patients, no matter how intractable the problems, no matter the obstacles. We offer children, adolescents, and adults realistic hope that they can have a better quality of life, whatever that might mean for them.

There is no disincentive for catapulting patients onto diagnostic odysseys. Our healthcare system incentivizes quantity of service over quality of care, short evaluations and Band-Aid solutions over comprehensive evaluations, and procedures over cognitive approaches. The system also favors the lowest-cost clinician by reimbursing providers the same, regardless of the experience of the clinician or the quality of care they can provide.

This is a brief catalog of problems hardwired into our healthcare delivery system. There is an obvious need for innovative solutions for delivering healthcare to special needs populations. Our organization fills this void. We continue to deliver dedicated care to our patients and their families while achieving measurable, beyond-the-norm results. We are a blueprint for the future of healthcare delivery, at least for neurological issues like autism and related disorders, the incidences of which have been steadily increasing for decades. We offer hope to many suffering families, perhaps like you, by providing optimized outcomes to patients of all ages.

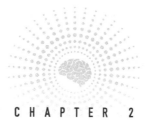

An Integrated Approach
That Works

You have probably heard of the formula $E=mc^2$. Albert Einstein's equation describing energy as a function of mass times the square of the speed of light is very possibly the most famous equation in the world. It is a cornerstone of his theory of special relativity, perhaps the most famous scientific theory in the world.

When Einstein proposed his theory at the turn of the twentieth century, it overturned human understanding of the universe, all of Newtonian physics, and other more far-fetched fields as well, including psychology and sociology. It reverberated in ordinary life because it offered a new perspective on literally everything.

The sociological effect of relativity was based on Einstein's ground-breaking assertion that motion and time were relative: they depended on where the observer was located and how fast they were moving. His analogy at the human level was an individual standing on a train moving forward at twenty miles per hour watching the adjacent train back out of the station at the same speed. The individual in question could be forgiven for believing their train was moving twice as fast as it was because their position relative to the other train was changing at forty miles per hour. An observer on the other train would come to a different conclusion—that their train was moving swiftly in reverse—based on the perspective from their vantage point. From the platform, a third observer would perceive each train moving at twenty miles per hour in opposite directions. Perception is a matter of perspective.

In fact, this is true in every aspect of life. Unquestionably, every one of us has encountered situations in which participants or observers of the same situation have had completely different reactions based on their own experiences, beliefs, education, psychology, and more.

Consider how graphic designers approach their work in email marketing: they know that bright colors and complex designs delight younger people and boost open rates while proving counterproductive when addressing older businesspeople.

> **Perception is a matter of perspective.**

For them, the formula for increased impact is simpler colors, shades of gray, and plenty of white space. They are responding to the same emailed design, with the same information, communicated through the same medium. Yet the chasm in perspective between individuals based on age and station in life spawns a similar chasm in their reaction to communicated materials.

In the movies, the altered realities of different perspectives are fodder for plot thickening and intrigue. Perspective can also affect diagnoses and treatment plans in healthcare, an insight often unnoticed by the industry itself. Specialists with vast expertise in a narrow topic can lose sight of the larger picture, while primary care providers may miss the telling details that require more specialized expertise. This can cause a profession to become sclerotic and resistant to innovation.

In our practice, populated by open-minded practitioners, we *invite* alternative points of view. We believe that our practice is serving its patients when we gather all the perspectives possible to consider each case individually. Our road map for diagnosis and treatment starts with an unusual number of evaluations and assessments, some of them overlapping but gathered through varying clinical prisms. This affords us the closest thing to a 360-degree view of the patient and their clinical profile and underlying biological mechanisms, indicating the clearest path forward in treatment.

THE NECESSARY EVALUATION JOURNEY

We start with the medical model of assessment. It begins with a neurological or neurodevelopmental specialist gathering clues from a patient's medical history that might suggest certain disorders and diseases. While analyzing this information, the specialist synthesizes what they learn with observational clues from an examination to detect abnormalities in the central and peripheral nervous system, as well as the body as a whole. This is the level of assessment most common at any practice level. It is important and necessary but merely one step on the assessment journey in our practice.

The foundation of our evaluation and assessment process is to gather an array of objective and subjective data and information that can be synthesized and translated into a useful and pragmatic diagnostic and treatment plan. The perspective of the neuropsychologist is a key piece to the diagnostic puzzle. Neuropsychologists use empirical and standardized testing instruments that can measure and quantify cognitive function and output: memory, executive function, intellectual levels, visual-spatial relationships, auditory and other sensory perceptions, academic achievement, and personality. Such information is vital for understanding the brain's baseline functional capacity and abilities, contributing to diagnostic formulations, and detecting neurocognitive changes over time from the natural history of a disorder or the effectiveness of treatment interventions.

Advanced office-based technologies can also play an important role in measuring the brain's function and output. Such instruments can tell us about brain activities that may not be observable. I have mentioned previously the high-density EEG tests we do that are patient friendly and more revealing than ordinary EEGs. Our HD-EEG tests assess the electrical activity of brain cells (neurons) and networks, which can provide information about brain function and structure and can be related to abnormalities such as seizures and alterations in awareness and attention. Such neurophysiological information can inform and alter clinical management.

Abnormal and problematic behavior might be a manifestation of underlying neurological problems, but it can also result from emotional or environmental incidents and influences or, in some cases, both mechanisms. However, behaviors are usually defined subjectively. This can lead to poor outcomes because of a number of factors: a poor understanding if there are identifiable reasons for triggering a difficult behavior, such as seeking attention or avoiding a task or demand, or if the behavior is biologically driven and not fully in the control of the individual; inability to understand the intensity and severity of problem behaviors; poor understanding of how behaviors interfere with daily functioning; and a lack of objective information concerning the impact of treatments. This is where our team of behavior analysts and therapists provides an important perspective and dimension to our comprehensive evaluations. By performing a "functional behavior analysis," we can determine functions of behaviors. For example, if a child with autism is found to be aggressive because they are seeking attention, behavioral management with a goal of reshaping this behavior can be successful and avoid treatments such as medications.

I'll share a real-life example of a child with a common clinical presentation we often see who benefited from our rigorous assessment protocol. Zach (not his real name) was four years old when he arrived in our offices with issues of inattention, anxiety, and mild developmental and behavioral challenges. This presented itself, in part, in episodic eye rolls, head bobs, and glassy-eyed stares. If you saw Zach, you might think he was spacing out or was disconnected with the world around him. As you can imagine, this was both frustrating and frightening for his parents, who feared for his future and yearned for the ordinary responses that parents cherish from their children.

Exposing Zach to a comprehensive evaluation helped us determine not only that he had mild autism spectrum disorder (previously called Asperger syndrome) but also a complicating factor that would ordinarily be difficult to detect—periodic subclinical seizures that were triggering his behavioral quirks and deflecting his attention from his environment and the people in it. We found these spikes of electrical activity in his brain using a state-of-the-art high-density EEG machine, situated in our office and employed in many of our clinical assessments.

Responding to the symptoms and causes rather than the diagnosis, we immediately treated Zach with a well-tolerated antiseizure medication. Drugs are not always the best answer or even an answer at all; sometimes they are just a shorthand response that is fast and convenient, even if they create negative side effects down the line. But in this case, we suspected that the medication prescribed, specifically targeting Zach's abnormal brain function and presenting few side effects, was the correct choice for this particular patient.

It turned out to be a good call. Zach exhibited "monumental" improvement, according to his mother, in attention and focus, as well as his behavioral issues. The eye rolling, head bobbing, and spacing out resolved almost immediately. This is one of those rare instances when prescribing an easily tolerated drug can produce the intended results without complications.

Zach's family was required to seek a second opinion, and he was admitted to the hospital for a twenty-four-hour conventional EEG study. Although it detected some of the same subclinical spikes that we found distorting Zach's behavior, hospital staff saw no clinical correlation of these electrical discharges with his symptoms. A neurologist recommended the discontinuation of his medication, which was all but curing the issue.

You can probably write the rest of this true story yourself. Zach's behavior immediately regressed to its previous state, undoing all the progress we had made. It didn't take long for the family to return to us for a reboot of his regimen, with a return to the same improved state.

What this story illustrates is the critical importance of that first, often perfunctory, step: comprehensive evaluation. The more complete the understanding of underlying issues instigating medical, neurological, and behavioral symptoms, the more effective the treatment plan is likely to be. This is analogous to a car care professional diagnosing a fluid leak beneath the engine as coolant loss and responding by adding coolant to your reservoir. If the actual problem is an oil leak, that treatment, no matter how expertly applied, will not address the issue at hand.

It is important to note that Zach's treatment transcended prescribing a pill for seizures. We also offered him therapy for social and anxiety issues related to his mild autism and have seen him make remarkable progress. His journey with us has been so successful largely as a result of the comprehensive and collaborative—you might even say obsessively so—assessment we conduct before diagnosing and treating.

Our integrated evaluation and assessment model is based upon two fundamental pillars: (1) identifying and determining the biological causes and contributions to diagnoses, symptoms, and signs, (2) and developing an extensive, objective, qualitative, and quantitative clinical profile of neurological, neuropsychological, neuropsychiatric, and behavioral functioning. We use advanced testing methodologies and technologies that can measure brain function, like the HD-EEG of the brain that Zach received, or a comprehensive neuropsychological evaluation, which together provide an overall clinical profile and biological basis to determine what is happening (or has happened) and why. Each of these methods of investigation alone is necessary yet insufficient to establish a 360-degree view of the individual patient's pathologies and strengths.

As we stress, we are diagnosis agnostic: the name of the condition does not determine our assessment or treatment, lest we narrow the scope of our understanding. We treat each patient individually based on their specific assessment, irrespective of the label or diagnostic code. That is how we found the subclinical electrical activity in Charlie's brain mentioned in the first chapter, which was causing him miniseizures unrelated to his mild autism spectrum disorder diagnosis. Absent that step, Charlie's progress would have always been hindered by an undetected and untreated mechanism in his brain. As it turned out, that was easily corrected and now poses no issue for him.

This protocol can be demonstrated through the visit of a hypothetical patient who comes to us for the first time. The neurologist (or other physician specialist, such as developmental-behavioral pediatrician) would examine their medical history and records first to establish a baseline of information and then discuss with the patient their reason for the visit. For example, a patient who presents with a headache would be asked about its severity, triggers, location, first onset, and so on. The neurologist and patient (or, in the cases of children, who comprise the majority of our patients, the parents) would discuss background issues like a history of head trauma and concussions, other illnesses and problems, family history of headaches or migraines, the use of medications and supplements, and more. The neurologist would delve deeply into the patient's history, considering developmental issues such as when they first began walking and talking, and observe involuntary movements like tremors and tics. All of this helps build a narrative about the patient.

As you are no doubt know, the pediatric neurologist will ask about the patient's family history, which can provide a deep well of clues. If an uncle has autism, for example, that offers a clue about a potential genetic basis for autism in a child. We cover the physical, cognitive, emotional, and psychological elements to the extent that patients or families can provide this kind of information because it represents important pieces of the larger puzzle. Once we understand the full environmental, biological, medical, developmental, educational, and genetic history of the patient, we can begin to weave a story of the person sitting across from us.

I should mention that in a practice like ours, in which many of the patients are pediatric, a majority of these discussions take place with the parent or some other surrogate. We do attempt to engage the patients themselves, no matter how young, to the extent practicable, in part so that they feel valued and heard. Additionally, there is a danger in total reliance on a third party. For example, we could discuss with parents and teachers the case of an eight-year-old boy who has ADHD and treat him with pharmaceuticals based on their testimony. If we objectively test him ourselves, we might discover that his problem is not ADHD but something else that leads to similar behavior, like a learning or sleep disorder, that would not be improved significantly by drugs.

Does all this create a diagnosis? Yes, but it is the biological phenotype and clinical profile that drive our precision treatment. (Note: The clinical phenotype is the overall description of an individual based on their observable physical features, developmental level, cognitive functioning, behavioral manifestations, and clinical findings. The biological phenotype refers to the observed or measured genetic, biochemical, and physiological properties causing or contributing to the overall clinical phenotype.)

We are not only interested in diagnoses, and the hypothetical case of the eight-year-old boy just mentioned demonstrates why. Our neurological/neurodevelopmental assessment generates a narrative of the particular individual sitting in front of the physician, with their own unique lifestyle, history, family dynamic, genetic makeup, and set of symptoms. Each person has their own unique story. What works for one individual with a particular condition might not for another with the same condition, so we take a more holistic view of the patient than simply boiling them down to a diagnosis. This does not suggest that there are not standard treatments for many conditions; it simply provides us with a deeper understanding of the possible variations among patients that must be considered when developing a treatment plan.

How unusual is the focus on narrative rather than diagnosis? Increasingly so. The growth of digital medicine, which is ubiquitous at this point, has replaced the account of each patient's life with a series of checked boxes, as if a human being is their strep throat. Prior to the hegemony of digital record keeping, I always spent most of my time on the handwritten notes whenever I reviewed the chart of a patient who had been seen by other clinicians. It provided more insight into who the patient was, as opposed to what their symptoms were.

This is where most evaluations end. For us, it is often the end of the beginning. In many cases, the neurologist discusses his or her preliminary findings with the rest of the multidisciplinary team to establish a possible course of treatment, recognizing that further testing and evaluation will be necessary to confirm, amend, or disprove the neurologist's conclusions. For a three-year-old child with autism, the neuropsychology team would conduct an empirically validated test for autism and an interview with the family to determine the level of severity of the condition. The behavior team would be consulted to determine whether there is a trigger to the child's behavior, biological drivers, or some other initiator, such as when a child learns to use bad behavior to get attention.

It is often appropriate for us to conduct genetic testing to discover genetic variants causing problems. Far more often than not, when our medical geneticist reanalyzes the genetic sequencing information, actionable information is found that eludes the grasp of the reporting laboratories. These noninvasive genetic tests—needing only a saliva sample—reveal a vast array of information otherwise hidden from the view of the neurologist and can significantly alter clinical management.

The assessment may not stop there. Abraham Lincoln said that if he had eight hours to chop down a tree, he would spend six of them sharpening his ax. We consider the extended process of evaluation a long-term investment in the treatment and health of our patients. A month of extended assessment could have prevented the decade-long diagnostic odyssey that Bobbi in chapter 1 endured, complete with repeated hospitalizations and more or less continuous misery. We recognize that patients are left waiting for answers during this meticulous and iterative process, but it bears fruit so often that failing to do so would be a disservice to our patients. We ask our patients, and often their parents, to trust that we are acting in their best interest. Most of them eventually come to see the efficacy of our methods.

In cases that warrant it, we will conduct an HD-EEG of the brain, like the one we used on four-year-old Zach. The cutting-edge equipment we use is patient friendly and significantly more illuminating than a conventional EEG you might get at a hospital. We might also recommend getting a blood sample for finding other potential medical causes or contributions to the presenting problems. Blood tests can have identifying markers of functional abnormalities of hormonal, renal, liver, immunological, and other systems. Subject to presenting findings, additional specialty evaluations, such as gastroenterology, cardiology, ophthalmology/developmental optometry, immunology, and others, may be indicated. Depending on a patient's presenting issues and symptoms or on the clues of the evaluation or other investigations, there are many other diagnostic tests that are considered. In the words of Alexander Graham Bell, "Before anything else, preparation is the key to success."

Only after we have gathered this plethora of data of objective and subjective information do we develop a treatment plan. This may also entail a multidisciplinary team conference. For an autism patient, it generally includes a review with the family of the findings and diagnostic implications and recommendations for therapeutic strategies, such as behavior management, medicines or nutrient supplements, guidance for proper sleep, and lifestyle changes. Some patients may require additional therapies, such as occupational therapy, speech-language therapy, or physical therapy, all of which are generally provided in school. Overall, our clinical model provides for a comprehensive, one-stop shop "under one roof" for assessment and treatment for neurological and neurodevelopmental issues.

A nonverbal eight-year-old boy with autism (we'll call him Max) came to our attention recently. He was already under the care of a primary care physician and a psychiatrist, along with behavioral supports in school. He exhibited a variety of behaviors of concern, including aggression, destructiveness, meltdowns, and self-injury. His doctors had him on a relatively high-dose cocktail of three medications: the stimulant Adderall, the antipsychotic risperidone, and the antianxiety drug clonazepam. This is a fairly standard combination for children with these behaviors, despite their many side effects. In Max's case, the medication had caused insomnia and a weight gain sufficient to push him into the obesity category. For all that, the behaviors showed no signs of ebbing.

Our initial neurological evaluation determined that it was necessary to understand the function of the behaviors: why they were occurring and what was setting them off. The behavior team analyzed how he presented while we simultaneously began to wean him from the medications because they were obviously ineffective and producing side effects. Our behavioral team initiated a functional behavior analysis in the child's home—his naturalistic setting—and found that the target behaviors were occurring to draw attention. Although the attention was negative (e.g., a reprimand), it was attention nonetheless and was inadvertently reinforcing and perpetuating his negative behaviors. The behavior team initiated parent training to recognize these behavior patterns and instituted reactions to these behaviors that included ignoring and redirection. Max's parents quickly caught on, and the severe behaviors subsided without the need for additional or alternative medications.

Despite the new and more effective behavior plan, Max remained prone to episodic behavioral escalations, verbal outbursts, hyper-activity, and agitation. Our neurologists found this fit a pattern of "autonomic over-responsivity" (i.e., poor regulation of behavioral and physiological responses to environmental stimulation). Additional testing included a high-density EEG, which uncovered "subclinical spikes" of electrical activity in the brain. Neurogenomic testing found a pathological variant in a gene that codes for a "calcium channel," which led to a hypothesis that Max's baseline maladaptive behaviors, severe behaviors, and sudden behavioral outbursts were triggered by "leaky" calcium channels on brain cells.

Our thinking was that once Max was "triggered" and his behaviors began to escalate, the resulting stress caused his defective calcium channels to allow sudden rushes of calcium into brain cells, further exacerbated by stress hormones, causing a chaotic and unregulated response, such as a "meltdown." In other words, a pathophysiological/biological process was overstimulating his brain and causing his disordered behavior. This information led to treatment with a medication that specifically blocked the calcium channel, and his behaviors improved. Simultaneously, we weaned Max off his other medications completely so that, eventually, he was taking one, beneficial medication, which also allowed him to lose weight.

This course of action is a treatment, not a cure. Max continued to require ongoing and educational interventions, but the ability to alleviate the severe behaviors made the situation more manageable for him and his family. It facilitated other behavioral and educational interventions, which reduced family stress and eliminated his destruction of the household. He is not cured, but nearly everything in his life is better, and for the first time, he is making progress toward becoming a more functional and independent young man.

MULTIDISCIPLINARY, INTERDISCIPLINARY, AND HOLISTIC APPROACHES

This is the advantage of employing an interdisciplinary and holistic approach to patient assessment, treatment, and care.

Before describing the advantage of this approach, I need to take a semantic detour. I've used "multidisciplinary" and "interdisciplinary" interchangeably, as many people do, but they are not precisely the same. A multidisciplinary approach brings together several fields of study to assess a problem and report their findings independently, with some synthesis of their results comprising the final determination. An interdisciplinary approach brings together those various disciplines to assess and analyze together in a significantly more integrated effort. Interdisciplinary approaches tend to be useful for novel symptom presentations but can be more chaotic and time consuming.

Come to think of it, our approach often transcends even "interdisciplinary" to occupy the space of "transdisciplinary," or at least that is our goal. A transdisciplinary method takes the collaborative aspect of an interdisciplinary approach to the next level, in which professionals not only work together in a symbiotic manner for the best interest of the patient but also do so with an understanding of every other professional's field of expertise.

In practice, at NeurAbilities our approach is variously multidisciplinary, interdisciplinary, and transdisciplinary, and some amalgam of the three. Most consequentially, irrespective of our assessment procedures, when the time comes to draw conclusions and develop a treatment plan, we are fully interdisciplinary in the sense that we invite all disciplines into the discussion. That is why, as I mentioned previously, the type of individuals we attract to our organization are more open-minded and creative thinkers willing to admit that they do not have all answers, and they practice in a setting in which the cultural values reinforce their perspective.

With this holistic approach, we have set out to create a home for people where they can get all their diagnostic and therapeutic services from one organization under one roof. We launched this healthcare organization almost two decades ago believing that our model of service delivery was valuable to patients, and the marketplace has validated that belief. The comprehensive services approach has been one-half of our success. The other half lies in our independence from the bureaucracy and confines of a large institution, like a hospital system. We have created a neurological medical home for our patients, and this has served them, and us, well.

THE SPECIALIST MEDICAL HOME

The concept of the medical home for primary care came to life in 1978, when a pediatrician in Hawaii created a comprehensive child health plan for children with special needs, establishing his office as the clearinghouse for information about each child and serving as gatekeeper for all the specialty care the children needed. Coordination of care for each child was managed at the physician's office in a system that connected all services through the doctor most knowledgeable about the patient's condition. The concept was premised on the theory that high-quality care and stronger doctor-patient relationships could keep patients healthier and out of expensive emergency rooms. It was first conceived as a strategy to deliver coordinated, comprehensive care to all children.

In the 1980s and '90s, as managed care grew to rein in costs, insurance companies viewed medical homes as an element in that strategy. In time, it appeared to many consumers that constraining costs had become the primary imperative of the medical home for insurers. Among their tactics to drive down overall healthcare expenses was providing incentives for gatekeeper physicians for reducing diagnostic testing, referrals, and the incidence of ER visits and hospital stays.

That concept lost favor as patients chafed at the strict rules governing their access to specialists and the irritant of clearing every specialist visit through their primary care practitioner's office. They rebelled against what they saw as the denial of care of HMOs (health maintenance organizations, which comprised the bulk of the early managed care plans) more focused on cost containment than on improving care. The anger over HMO-managed care was embodied in "drive-by deliveries," in which maternity wards were required to discharge mothers within twenty-four hours of uncomplicated deliveries. Rules like this fueled discontent about these arrangements and led to a stream of health insurance customers opting instead for preferred provider organizations with higher premiums but fewer constraints.

What was clear to us was that the medical home per se was not the issue; it never lost its effectiveness and efficiency. A study in 2004 found that widespread implementation of patient-centered medical homes would have improved overall health and reduced health disparities with concomitant reductions in healthcare costs of $67 billion annually.[21]

When we imported the patient-centered/family-centered medical home model to our office for specialty care, we attempted to retain its efficacy while upholding our patient and family focus. The special needs population that we see spends significantly more time in our office for tests, therapy, and follow-up than they do with their primary care provider, and our relationship with them is often long term. It makes sense for our office to serve as their principal care provider, particularly considering our comprehensive and holistic approach, which ensures that many of the specialty care services our patients will need are provided in the same practice.

We should be clear that we are not primary care providers, who typically serve as the medical home for primary care. We instead manage the specialty care of patients who receive the bulk of their healthcare from specialists while communicating and coordinating with their primary care providers as "neighbors."

---

21   William R. Phillips, "Editorial: Research in the Community and Clinic," *Annals of Family Medicine* 2, no. 2 (2004): 98–100, doi:10.1370/afm.129.

Additionally, because specialists are less common and farther apart than primary care physicians, tending to be more regional than local, patients and families are willing to travel for our services—even over two hours away. To lessen this burden, we have opened more regional facilities and also have introduced telemedicine. Primary care physicians treating these patients are more likely to wait until problems arise to refer them for neurological treatment, despite empirical evidence that prevention is a better—and less expensive—strategy. As a Specialty Care Medical Home, we capture patients earlier in the process but continue to work with primary care providers.

The advantage of being an independent operation untethered from a large institution is salient in these instances. A hospital system has a vested interest in referring patients to providers whose practices are owned by the system or are at least part of their network. They are loath to refer patients outside the system, even for services not provided within. Because we are beholden to no one, we can work with any kind of provider anywhere. We keep internal all the specialty care we provide but refer patients regularly for services not under our roof. This addresses a major complaint of families—the fragmentation of care.

Hospital systems, despite their horizontal integration across many specialties, manage paradoxically to fragment care with their complex bureaucracies even as they bring providers together under one umbrella. Many of our patients receive all the services they need in our office—and perhaps at home or school—and even those who require outside interventions know that their care is coordinated in our office and communication about their case is continual.

The impetus for our medical home concept has nothing to do with insurance company profits; we are focused on providing effective, compassionate, individualized care. A serendipitous side effect of this model is the way defragmentation of service saves the healthcare system tremendous sums of money through reduced hospitalizations, ER visits, and testing utilization. It requires an enlightened view of the process to understand the cost-saving aspect of this model because it is expensive up front to do testing at the level of comprehensiveness that we do, but it saves resources in the long run. Had a provider thought of conducting comprehensive but targeted tests on Bobbi at the beginning of her ten-year healthcare odyssey, much of her pain and suffering might have been averted.

For patients and their families, our medical home concept offers convenience, expedited diagnosis, treatment, continuity of care across the life span, and peace of mind.

Sandy and Tony have seven children in a blended family, four of whom have special needs. Their daughter Lexi is a patient with us, and we serve as her medical home. She has seen a diversity of specialists under our one roof—neuropsychologists, genetic testing, ABA therapy, and more. It has been a godsend for her parents.

"It's getting your diagnoses and all the pieces that need to be clinched together. Whether it be child study teams, performed care, guardianship, or DDD applications, I never worry about asking NeurAbilities how I can get the proper information that is going to help me be successful in my daughter's journey. They understand that it is something we need and help us get it," Sandy told us.

"Sometimes you will go to another practitioner and, they'll say, 'Well, you need to talk to this (other) practitioner'—and then you're waiting three to six months to get another appointment, whereas with NeurAbilities, you are already in the system; you are an established patient, and they just plug you right in," Tony added.

"Fee-for-service" is the predominant system of paying healthcare providers for services rendered. However, such a system incentivizes volume (generating more office visits or medical procedures) rather than value. Government and commercial insurance payers are looking for better solutions that control costs while maintaining the integrity of quality outcomes. Often referred to as "advanced alternative payment models," our Specialty Care Medical Home concept is in line with such innovative reimbursement models by addressing the main drivers of healthcare costs and poor outcomes for special needs populations—namely, fragmentation of care, overuse of pharmaceuticals, overutilization of hospital-based resources, poor accessibility to specialists, inefficient continuity of care, and lack of life-span services.

Our patient George is a living example of that. He started having epileptic seizures multiple times every day at age eleven. His mother says it became such a normal part of his life that he would stop mid-sentence, experience a small seizure, and then finish the sentence. Understandably, his mother was resigned to the idea that her son could never have a normal life.

When George was brought to us, we began serving as his Specialty Care Medical Home. After all, the seizures were the central focus of his daily life. It made no sense for his primary care practitioner, who could do little for his seizures, to organize his care. We coordinated his sleep studies, EEGs, medications, and a variety of clinical providers and ensured that all that disparate care was integrated into one patient experience.

George actually talks about our office as *home*: "This is the place that makes me feel at home," he says. Better yet, George's life improved from seizure-dominated to seizure-punctuated to relative seizure freedom. George is gainfully employed today, and I was honored to attend his wedding, an event neither he nor his mother could have dreamed would ever take place.

PRECISION OR PERSONALIZED MEDICINE

When you go to the bakery to pick up a cake for your daughter's ninth birthday, you can choose a ready-made cake if you like. It is designed for the average child, with the ingredients most children like in cake and decorated the way an average child might like. That is fine if your daughter likes the ingredients chosen by someone else and the generic message written in icing at the top wishing the recipient a happy birthday.

But suppose your daughter is not really a fan of chocolate or loves *The Little Mermaid* or would be excited to see her name on it. The one-size-fits-all cake will elicit a tepid response from your child because your child is an individual, not a cohort.

In that case, you order a custom-made cake because any decent bakery makes cakes to order if they plan to remain in business long. People of all ages like their cakes personalized. The cake you bring home is vanilla and strawberry, includes "Happy Birthday" with her name written in icing, and includes a depiction, also in icing, of the Little Mermaid herself. The cake, personalized to the desires of your precious child, will be a much bigger hit with her than the generic version would be.

The benefit of customized service that recognizes the recipient's uniqueness is obvious in the case of a nine-year-old girl's smile. Multiply that by its benefits when applied to the care of patients in a healthcare setting, when life or death—or at least long-term health—is at stake, and the imperative to provide services this way becomes overwhelming.

The National Institutes of Health's Precision Medicine Initiative describes personalized or precision medicine as "an emerging approach for disease treatment and prevention that takes into account individual variability in genes, environment, and lifestyle for each person."[22]

---

22 "Precision Medicine," NIH Office of Logistics and Acquisition Operations, 2016, https://olao.od.nih.gov/content/precision-medicine.

Disease prevention and treatment strategies developed for the average person are woefully inadequate when applied to unique individuals whose differences may be consequential to their care. This is not a new concept. For example, no hospital would transfuse "average" blood into a patient; that could lead to rejection or death. Instead, they take great care to ascertain the patient's blood type and transfuse only the compatible types into each individual patient.

Unfortunately, this is the exception in medicine, rather than the rule. The ibuprofen bottle in your medicine cabinet recommends the consumption of one or two two-hundred-milligram pills every four to six hours for pain without knowing a host of variables like your body weight. A 250-pound man likely requires a larger dose than a hundred-pound woman, even before accounting for other variables like metabolism or genetics.

Embedded in our mantra that we are diagnosis agnostic, that we treat the underlying biological causes and contributions of symptoms and behaviors, is the practice of precision medicine. By eschewing diagnostic labels and instead defining clinical manifestations and then performing comprehensive diagnostic testing to identify biological mechanisms, we can home in on specific causes and targeted therapies, rather than fall back on what works adequately "on average."

Our primary method of establishing an individualized diagnosis and care plan is through clinical profiling and biological phenotyping. Phenotyping often refers to outward observable or measurable characteristics or traits arising from a person's genetic makeup and the interaction of their genes with the environment, whereas we refer to *biological phenotyping* (or subphenotyping) to mean identifying and defining various biological (genetic, metabolic, electrophysiologic, and many more) causes and contributions to the physical phenotype.

Clinical profiling refers to the various measures and observations of brain and body function. Biology does not respect a diagnosis, as we could be blind to a patient's diagnosis and still create an individual profile of that person if we know their underlying biological phenotype and clinical profile.

For example, as we have discussed previously, rather than respond to a general diagnosis of ADHD by prescribing some drug or another—which is the common procedure in medicine today—we might find subclinical spikes on HD-EEG, suggesting treatment that is focused on spike suppression with improvements in attention. Employing this kind of personalization of diagnosis and treatment has spillover effects for other members of the family who may share genetic traits.

How does a small, specialized practice like ours operate at a high-tech level on par or better than what is offered through multibillion-dollar hospital systems? This goes back to our independence and agility. We are not beholden to the complex bureaucracies of large institutions; instead, we can pivot quickly when conditions require and offer our patients a level of targeted efficiency that is hard to match. We can be nimble and creative, responding to new ideas as quickly as the next day, whereas it might take months to years at a large, bureaucratic enterprise.

Understanding neurodevelopmental and neuropsychiatric disorders from the biological and clinical perspective, rather than merely from the observable externalizing findings, is the future of medicine, one we have been practicing for almost two decades. Where most healthcare providers focus on the suppression of symptoms and behaviors, we have been digging deeper with an approach that informs a more precise approach to treatment. Being ahead of the curve has allowed us to refine that process and bring it to a higher level. We have changed a paradigm that long ago required overhauling and even now remains the dominant method of diagnosis and treatment.

Our patients deserve better, and that is what they get. The problem is, all patients deserve better, and if they are not receiving treatment from a tiny handful of practices like ours that are independent, comprehensive, and customized, they may not be getting it. We want all patients with neurological disorders to receive the high level of care we provide, irrespective of whether we are the providers of that care.

DOES AUTISM EXIST?

I gave a lecture a few years ago to a group of behavior analysts in which I questioned whether autism existed in the way it has been generally defined and diagnosed as a behavioral disorder. I don't actually mean to minimize the terrible toll that this spectrum of disorders has inflicted on millions of families. It is a source of pain for many families, and I applaud everyone involved in the struggle to help those with autism spectrum disorder live happy, independent lives. And that is quite the point.

In this way, my argument was that autism should be diagnosed and managed from a biological model, like cancer. Any researcher in the oncology field can testify that they are not working with cancer but with a specific disease unlike any others. Cancer—unregulated cell growth—is an umbrella term used to describe an array of diseases that work differently, each with a unique damage signature, each wreaking a distinct brand of havoc at the cellular level. Most cancers form tumors—large, localized collections of cancer cells—but leukemia and other blood cancers generally do not. Some cancers metastasize rapidly, most notably pancreatic cancer, but others, like some forms of prostate cancer, take an exceptionally long time to grow or spread. (Even then, some forms of prostate cancer are more aggressive and can spread rapidly, demonstrating that even within forms of cancer there are variations that can mean the difference between life and death.) Some cancers appear to have a strong genetic component, like breast cancer, while others, like lung cancer, appear to have a significant environmental etiology. And so on.

Because cancer is not a single disease, it cannot be addressed with a uniform treatment plan. There are different types of biological subtypes of cancer that can be traced all the way to a genetic level, which offers clues about the proper treatment. The choice of treatment may depend on various factors, including the organ of origin, the degree of cellular spread, the type of cells as seen under the microscope, and in some cancers, their genetic signatures, as well as many other factors. Thus, the "biological phenotype" along with the "clinical profile" will lead to precision, and more effective treatments. Why can't autism be diagnosed and treated with a similar biological or medical model?

In other words, a focus on precision medicine has created powerful new tools to fight some cancers in some people by tailoring the treatment to the unique genetic makeup and other biological features of the individual. This is exactly the approach we take to neurological and neurodevelopmental disorders, and why I titled my talk "Does Autism Exist?"

The approach that medical science has taken in the ongoing fight against cancer should be exported to developmental and behavioral disorders. There is precious little research identifying the biological component of autism. We have myriad classifications within autism that fail to reveal anything about the source of the disorder itself or of its many symptoms, like seizures.

Yet given the immense clinical and etiological variability among individuals with autism spectrum disorder diagnoses, it should be clear to anyone in the field who is paying attention that precision medicine offers the most opportunity for advancement in the field. Indeed, a study back in 2016 by two British researchers and a scientist at a Swiss pharmaceutical company drew this very conclusion and urged more research into the "multiple etiologies and pathophysiological mechanisms" that make "precision medicine the most promising approach to effective treatments for individuals with the overall umbrella condition."[23]

The diagnosis for most neuropsychiatric disorders, such as autism spectrum disorder, can be assigned regardless of the biological cause. Understanding the underlying biological phenotypes can provide more clinically useful information than only assigning a nonspecific name such as autism. A study by a group of researchers led by Thomas Frazier in the *Journal of the American Academy of Child & Adolescent Psychiatry* evaluating the validity of proposed *Diagnostic and Statistical Manual of Mental Disorders*, fifth edition criteria for autism spectrum disorder proposed the same thing a decade ago. "Neurobiological studies will be useful for determining ... whether the DSM-5 ASD diagnosis can be empirically parsed into biologically meaningful sub-phenotypes," they wrote.[24]

It has been said about virtually everything that if you want to know why people do the things they do, just follow the money. In the next chapter, we will delve into the role cost plays in the delivery of care to patients with neurological disorders. Cost is a huge component of healthcare, but, as you'll soon see, when everybody is focused on up-front cost, they may not realize that quality doesn't have to be more expensive. Indeed, we can demonstrate that just the opposite is true: the more decisions are made purely to trim up-front costs, the more expensive they end up being.

---

23   Eva Loth et al., "Defining Precision Medicine Approaches to Autism Spectrum Disorders: Concepts and Challenges," *Frontiers in Psychiatry* 7 (November 29, 2016): 188, https://doi.org/10.3389/fpsyt.2016.00188.

24   Thomas Frazier et al., "Validation of Proposed DSM-5 Criteria for Autism Spectrum Disorder," *Journal of the American Academy of Child and Adolescent Psychiatry* 51 (2012): 28–40.e3, doi: 10.1016/j.jaac.2011.09.021.

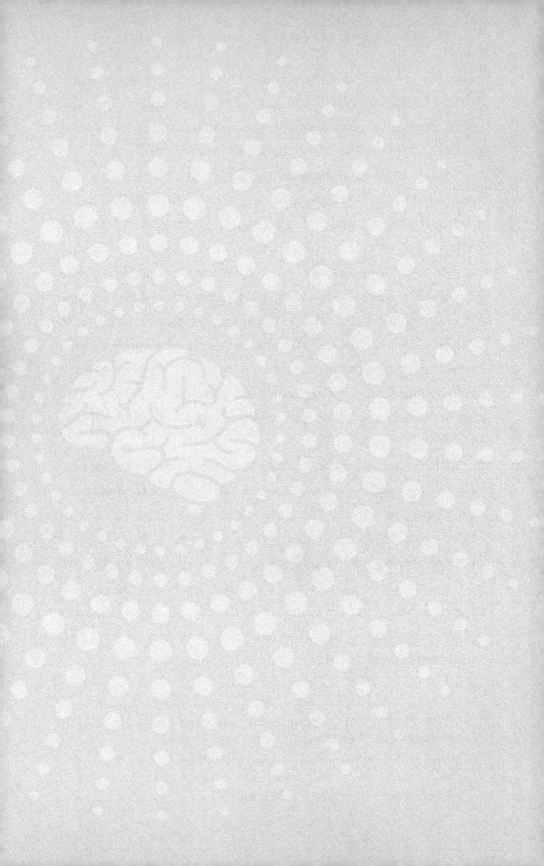

Cheaper Isn't Always Less Expensive

When Evan's son Chris was born, she knew immediately something was wrong. Seeing his behavior as a young child, that might not have been quite as hard to believe, but the only explanation for this at the time of his birth is mother's intuition, for which there is no scientific substitute. Mothers often intuit things about their children that physicians and other people of science can only, at best, later confirm. This was one such case.

It did not take long for Evan's gut feeling to make itself evident in Chris. At an early age he was diagnosed with autism.

Study after study has demonstrated that the earlier a child can be diagnosed with autism, the earlier appropriate treatment can begin and the more time is available to help the child learn strategies to manage the most problematic elements of the condition and adapt to the neurotypical world around them. This is because, in part, a baby's brain is a learning machine, establishing the neural connections that will lead to a lifetime of learning. From infancy through about year three, children are building the synaptic connections that will last their entire lives and allow them to grasp language, interpret sensory stimulation, and do all the things that humans do. In almost every category of human development, the first five or so years of life are critical.

Thus, an early diagnosis should have been a boon to Chris and his future development. In his case, however, it was a double-edged sword. Chris became his diagnosis in the eyes of his doctors and his school, and all his treatment was focused on the one aspect of him, as if a human being is simply a single diagnosis, rather than a complicated being that can be many things at once. (As Walt Whitman wrote, "Do I contradict myself? Very well then, I contradict myself. I am large; I contain multitudes.") Chris was more than a single diagnosis, and before long he began exhibiting behaviors that did not fit into the autism rubric.

In a siloed, fee-for-service healthcare system, it made sense to treat Chris through the single lens of autism. Healthcare practitioners with their specific areas of expertise would be reimbursed for creating a diagnosis and treating it using the best practices available, irrespective of the efficacy of that care. A healthcare practitioner trained to treat autism will treat autism where they see it. As the old saying goes, if your only tool is a hammer, every problem looks like a nail.

In fact, even if a practitioner suspected that autism was not the entirety of Chris's conditions, they had little incentive to dig deeper. Whatever else might be determined about Chris would require intervention by another specialist at a different practice and complicate his care without any remuneration for the original clinical practice. The siloed healthcare system disincentivizes further investigation.

In *All the President's Men*, the movie account of the *Washington Post* exposé about the 1972 Watergate scandal, the anonymous source, "Deep Throat," tells Bob Woodward and Carl Bernstein that if they wanted to get to the heart of the matter, they needed to "follow the money." This advice is adaptable to understanding a wide variety human endeavors, as true in healthcare as it is in politics and criminal activity. If you want to know why healthcare delivery is irrationally fragmented, follow the money.

The money in the healthcare system encourages disjointed, siloed activity. Funding mechanisms do not exist to encourage coordinated care from experts in a variety of disciplines and with a variety of perspectives in a single "medical home." The fact that Evan and her family could not get answers about Chris's condition beyond autism is not surprising; indeed, it would have been surprising if they had, given the state of our healthcare system. In defense of the physicians and other healthcare providers with whom her family was working, they were simply acting as the system encouraged them to act.

Chris and his mom eventually found their way to our practice, frustrated by the lack of progress he was making despite the early autism diagnosis and the intensive treatment he was receiving. As I have said, we are diagnosis agnostic; that is, we don't look at a patient's diagnosis but at their clinical symptoms and signs, obtain further neurodiagnostic information, and then determine a plan of care based on the patient's clinical profile and biological subgrouping (subphenotype).

Ultimately, it doesn't matter what label we apply to a patient because every patient is different, and biological lyand neurologically diverse. Even within autism, we talk about "the spectrum," because children fall on a long continuum of conditions, and even within that continuum, each child exhibits their condition differently—just as all of us have our own personal characteristics.

Imagine two people you would describe as introverts; you don't mean they are the same in every way and have the same predilections, behaviors, or interests. It is simply a convenient label you have applied to two people to distinguish them from extroverts but little else. You wouldn't assume that because both people are introverts that they both react to frustration, or being insulted, or getting their favorite food exactly the same way, would you?

In Chris's case, we saw behaviors that raised questions clearly not answered by a simple autism diagnosis. We ran a series of tests, including HD-EEGs that found unusual brain wave activity. We ran genetic tests that uncovered a rare genetic disorder. That led to the development of a treatment plan based, not on a behavioral diagnosis or the narrow expertise of a single practitioner, but on the underlying biology based on overwhelming evidence from a comprehensive diagnostic workup and analysis by a collaborative team of practitioners from multiple disciplines. By performing a comprehensive diagnostic evaluation and neurodiagnostic testing, we can provide targeted and effective therapies based on our findings. Being able to provide comprehensive evaluations and treatment interventions within one place is convenient, efficacious, and cost-effective. This may appear as more "expensive," but it is overall less costly by elimi-

> **Ultimately, it doesn't matter what label we apply to a patient because every patient is different, and biologically and neurologically diverse. Even within autism, we talk about "the spectrum," because children fall on a long continuum of conditions, and even within that continuum, each child exhibits their condition differently—just as all of us have our own personal characteristics.**

nating other expensive and unnecessary testing. Effective treatments avoid additional issues and problems that lead to excessive expense.

"Thank goodness he wasn't pigeonholed as just autistic," said Evan's mom. "Because it turns out that's a small piece of him, but that's not all of him. I can't describe in words how valuable that information is to us."

This is the way a healthcare system should work, and would work, if reimbursement were based on the value of services provided to the patient, not simply on the amount of activity produced by a diagnosis without regard to actual outcomes. This kind of collaboration and coordination of care would be the norm if the reimbursement system reflected a coordinated, integrated, holistic approach to care, rather than on each individual practitioner contributing iteratively, as if patient care is the simple sum of disconnected nodes of treatment.

It's a bit of a tortured analogy, I acknowledge, but imagine this approach applied to an orchestra, where each musician is compensated for their virtuoso performance without regard for its relationship with the rest of the ensemble. The flutists demonstrate their brilliance on Rimsky-Korsakov's frenzied "Flight of the Bumblebee," while the violins show off their skill on Bartok's Violin Sonata. Meanwhile the saxophones are channeling the jazz stylings of Charlie Parker, while percussionists are pounding out African drumbeats. At the same time, the mezzo-soprano delivers the lyrical beauty of Verdi's *Aida* in a voice so crystalline she could shatter glass. Would the result be beautiful? Quite the contrary: It would be noise.

Each artist or group of artists might be performing at their peak separately, but musical scores require synergy among the instruments just as our physical, mental, emotional, and psychological processes must support each other. We contain multitudes that must be understood not only as discrete units but also as a single, functioning being. Our body and mind are, in many ways, an orchestra, with each performer playing their individual role in concert with the community of performers around them.

To be clear, this is not a problem of incompetent or uncaring practitioners. The majority of doctors, nurses, therapists, and other healthcare providers choose their profession because they care about others and are motivated intrinsically to help people. But they are individuals working within a system that dictates how they can act. This is a systemic problem that creates perverse incentives and disincentives for practitioners. These restrictions can inhibit critical and innovative thinking to the detriment of the provider and patient.

The renowned management consultant W. Edwards Deming discovered in the 1950s that in American businesses, particularly in large, bureaucratic companies, the primary job of managers was not to succeed but to avoid responsibility for failure. Deming had previously taken his theories and focus on quality to postwar Japan, spearheading that country's economic miracle from devastation to wealth in less than a generation. When he returned to the United States, he devised his Total Quality Management system based on fourteen simple tenets focused on quality and continuous improvement.

Deming understood that people want to do a good job, to be engaged in their work, and take pride in its quality, but they respond to the conditions around them. Where the system stresses quality as the primary imperative and company leadership supplies the tools to produce that quality, the company flourishes. Where activity is treasured over quality, where management doesn't lead but rules by fear, the system will produce the activity demanded, and each employee will most highly prize evading blame for anything that goes wrong. Deming's teachings took hold in the 1980s in the United States and helped usher in four decades of nearly uninterrupted prosperity.

The US healthcare system could use a dose of Dr. Deming, who lived a full life until his death in 1993. In healthcare, the classic physician-patient relationship has been twisted in such a way that the focus is on volume of service and treating disease, not on quality and disease prevention. The insurance fee-for-service system has turned healthcare into the delivery of widgets under the pretense it will be cost-effective. And the irony is, this focus on cost-effectiveness may very well be the most cost-*ineffective* model of all.

THE CURIOUS, TORTURED HISTORY OF AMERICAN HEALTHCARE

You might be wondering: *How?* How did we end up with a healthcare system that no one would create today if they were starting from scratch? The answer to that question goes all the way back to World War II, when wage and price controls were instituted to prevent profiteers from exploiting shortages resulting from resources being diverted to the war effort.

Unions, which represented five times as many private-sector employees in the early 1940s as they do today, worked around the wage caps by negotiating various benefits that had monetary value but were not considered pay. Primary among them was health insurance, back then a minuscule cost to employers and small benefit to employees.

Following the war, Americans across sectors began demanding the benefit of health insurance, to the point where it became a de facto part of employment, like vacation time and retirement savings. With the advent of Medicare in 1965, primarily for individuals aged sixty-five and older, and Medicaid, primarily for families living in poverty, the federal government got into the health insurance business. Current procedural terminology, or CPT codes, were developed by the American Medical Association (AMA) in 1966. These five-digit codes corresponded to a wide array of medical services and procedures provided by physicians and continue to be used to this day.

Through the ensuing 1960s and up to 1992, physicians charged a fee-for-service that could vary from practice to practice—and patient to patient—but was somewhat constrained by free-market competition and principles. Medicare brought some price uniformity to the system with a "customary, prevailing, and reasonable (CPR)" charge system. Commercial insurance companies developed fee schedules for what they would pay for services, using a similar system to Medicare ("usual, customary, and reasonable [UCR]"), but these insurance companies negotiated payments with physicians and hospitals. Physicians were able to balance bill patients or waive the portion of their fees not paid for by Medicare or commercial insurance. Additionally, the majority of physicians were in private, independent practices often on the medical staff of hospitals—often multiple hospitals—but not hospital employees. This fee-for-service reimbursement model reigned during this time for private practices. Although there existed many rules and regulations, physicians had greater independence, and there were fewer bureaucratic intrusions into their ability to practice medicine. Likewise, patients had greater choice of providers, and this free-market ability pushed providers to focus on quality of care and fair market fees. Although there were growing concerns about the costs of healthcare, very little was from physician payments; rather, hospitalizations, pharmaceuticals, end-of-life care, long-term care, and more constituted the primary drivers of higher costs.

In 1989, the Omnibus Budget Reconciliation Act of 1989 established a Medicare fee schedule, fixing what physicians could be paid by Medicare and eventually restricting physicians from balance-billing anything above these fees. The year 1992 was a watershed one in healthcare reimbursement systems. The resource-based relative value scale (RBRVS) was introduced by Medicare and fundamentally changed the way physician services were being paid. The federal government established a standardized physician RBRVS payment schedule based on resource costs, with a goal to stabilize payments. Commercial payers were not obligated to meet the Medicare initiatives but often will adopt them as a baseline for negotiating physician payments. In response to the RBRVS, the AMA created a system to assign relative value units (RVUs) to each CPT code based upon the costs to deliver the CPT service, such as physician work to deliver the service, office overhead, malpractice insurance costs, and geographic adjustments. Medicare has adopted the RVU system for CPT codes but assigns the dollar amount per RVU on a yearly basis.

Other forces during the final decades of the twentieth century and continuing into the twenty-first century greatly affected the practice of medicine. Managed care organizations emerged in the 1970s, such as health maintenance organizations (HMOs) and preferred provider organizations (PPOs), creating "gatekeepers" to limit involvement of specialists and reduce diagnostic testing, which created many restrictions for hospitalizations and surgeries. How? Payments to physicians were often capitated to global amounts per patient, so the fewer referrals or the less testing done, the greater the physician payment. Additionally, the concept of "preauthorization" was eventually introduced, whereby many procedures and medications are not covered by the insurance payer if not approved prior to disbursement, resulting in tremendous administrative burdens on physicians and their staff, as well as introducing delays in care. Patient copayments and coinsurance costs created further disincentive for utilization of healthcare services, sometimes to the detriment of patient health. Furthermore, patients could only access physicians within the managed care network, greatly restricting patient choice of practices.

Initially, many physicians were somewhat jaded and did not realize that managed care was a threat to their independence and way of practicing medicine. However, the growth of managed care was largely driven by the insurance companies' ability to contract employers and patients to their networks, eventually causing physicians to see their patient populations dwindle to the point they were forced to contract with the managed care organization or face closure of their practices. In response, there have been physician-led initiatives to counter managed care, or to provide better leverage for negotiation, via independent physician associations (IPAs), physician practice management companies (PPMCs), management services organizations (MSOs), accountable care organizations (ACOs), and more. All the while there have been major increases in rules and regulations governing the practice of medicine and tremendous rises in the costs of running a physician practice, such as intensive information technology (IT) hardware and software, electronic medical records (EMRs), billing and collection costs, compliance expenses, and much more, coupled with diminishing payments and reimbursements for services. The passage of the Affordable Care Act in 2010 also created adverse pressures on independent practices by further narrowing physician networks, choice, and practice options, and caused many patients to have to leave trusted physicians they had been seeing for years. For the consumer, even "in-network" insurance that is "affordable" can be unusable due to unaffordable deductibles and rate increases.

The net result has been a major shift of physicians to hospital/institutional employment and consolidation of private practices into large networks. Whereas small independent practices predominated in the mid-to-late twentieth century, they have become a minority.

Despite these monumental alterations in healthcare delivery and reimbursements, costs continue to rise for both government and commercial payers. The Kaiser Family Foundation (KFF) examined the sources of Medicare funding in 2018, finding that payroll taxes accounted for only 36 percent; the federal government's general fund, 43 percent; and premiums, a mere 15 percent. The remaining revenue came from transfers from states, Social Security benefit taxes, and earned interest. Statistics from 2018 from the Centers for Medicare & Medicaid Services (CMS), which is the agency that administers Medicare, paint a bleak picture:

- Medicare spending increased 6.4 percent to $750.2 billion, or 21 percent of total national health expenditures.

- Medicaid spending rose 3 percent to $597.4 billion, or 16 percent of total national health expenditures.

- Medicare average yearly spending growth is projected to be 7.4 percent for 2018 to 2027, which will exceed that of Medicaid and private health insurance.

Thus, have all these changes in our healthcare system been beneficial or effective? By determining payments based solely on costs (RVUs), the value of the service to patients is neglected. Thus, the people making the reimbursement rules implicitly acknowledge that the patient is not relevant to the healthcare system except as the table across which providers and insurers negotiate their rates. Furthermore, RVUs are divorced entirely from the outcome of the procedure. There is literally no accommodation in the reimbursement for the quality of service or the experience of the provider, and so, indirectly, the current billing system disincentivizes spending the time to produce better-quality results. Healthcare providers' productivity is being measured by volume without any consideration for the efficacy of the service, its outcome for the patient, or its sustainability. RVUs do not account for much of physician work that is needed to produce an optimized outcome, such as professional activity needed to maintain knowledge and expertise; teaching, mentoring, and supervision; preauthorizations and appeals with insurance companies; and administrative stress.

Physicians who work for hospitals or whose practices are owned by them—now over half of all physicians and growing—are contractually required to meet performance quotas based on "productivity" and utterly silent as to quality and other factors contributing to value. These and other factors are contributing to the alarmingly increased phenomena of physician fatigue and burnout. "Burnout" among physicians is an increasingly recognized condition, and not only is detrimental to the physician's health, but will secondarily affect patient care. Physician burnout is often characterized by emotional exhaustion, feelings of cynicism and detachment, and a sense of ineffectiveness at work with a low sense of personal accomplishment.[25]

I have been fortunate to have explored these issues as a member of key task forces with a group of eminent professional colleagues. Essentially the groups concluded there is an urgent need for the recognition of the value a child neurologist provides to patients, health systems, and medical schools. If not addressed urgently, the present critical shortage of child neurologists will worsen, and the workforce will not be able to meet the demand for child neurology services in this country.[26, 27, 28]

25 Neil Busis et al., "Burnout, Career Satisfaction, and Well-Being among US Neurologists in 2016," *Neurology* 88 (2017): 1–12, doi: 10.1212/WNL.0000000000003640.

26 Peter Kang et al., "The Child Neurology Clinical Workforce in 2015: Report of the AAP/CNS Joint Taskforce," *Neurology* 87 (2016): 1384–1392, doi: 10.1212/WNL.0000000000003147.

27 Donald Gilbert et al., "Child Neurology Recruitment and Training: Views of the Residents and Child Neurologists from the 2015 AAP/CNS Workforce Survey," *Pediatric Neurology* 66 (2016): 89–95. doi: 10.1016/j.pediatrneurol.2016.08.018.

28 Mary Zupanc et al., "Child Neurology in the 21st Century: More Than the Sum of Our RVUs," *Neurology* 94, no. 2 (2020): 75–82, doi: 10.1212/WNL.0000000000008784.

If this sounds like the complaint of an individual practitioner, consider this: not only does the insurance payment model—government or commercial—not support good practice and optimized patient outcomes, but it also costs Americans hundreds of billions of dollars annually through taxes and premiums. Insurance adds tremendous complexity and expense to the system—doubling the cost of healthcare, according to some estimates. It creates a massive layer of administrative costs to providers merely to deal with the dozens of insurance carriers connected with patients. Consider the case of one urgent care center in a small city: the facility had to work with more than six hundred insurance company plans with dozens of different claims processes. It had to write contracts with six hundred different plans and credential all its physicians and physician's assistants and nurse practitioners with six hundred plans. It had to audit its billing for six hundred different plans, defend its charges to six hundred plans, and attempt to collect payment from six hundred different plans. The insurance operation consumed more costs than all the patient care the company delivered. The CEO eventually quit the company to found a new urgent care model that can charge half as much because it doesn't contract insurance payers.

There is also the issue of facility versus nonfacility reimbursement: government and commercial insurers will pay a higher amount to a hospital ("facility") than to a nonfacility for the same service (CPT code). Thus, independent organizations like ours can provide an equivalent service for less cost. The rationale for this is the higher overhead costs at hospitals, but it also suggests the value of private, independent healthcare organizations in providing better value at reduced costs.

In addition, insurers have a certain amount of incentive to deny payment for uncommon procedures, or demand preauthorizations or tiers of appeals that deter providers from pursuing approval, resulting in patients having to forgo important and valuable diagnostic procedures or medications.

We are not the first or only practitioners to recognize that the most effective healthcare practice delivers good outcomes that reduce the need for patients to return. Indeed, the notion dates to ancient China, where physicians were paid when patients got well, not when they were sick. We need to recall that one of the sacrosanct foundations and cornerstones of clinical medicine has been the doctor-patient relationship. In fact, there is scientific evidence that the relationship between patients and clinicians can improve health outcomes.[29]

However, the proverbial "consultation room" has been invaded by many others that are not necessarily working in the patient's or physician's best interests. These uninvited parties are lurking in the corners, under the desk, looking over shoulders, and hovering over the physician; they include insurance auditors and peer reviewers; CPT coders; bureaucrats; regulators; EMR manufacturers; pharma reps; healthcare economists; endless hospital, insurance, and license credentialing and recredentialing processes; internet and social media physician rating sites; and more: all affecting—often adversely—physician-patient interactions and physician autonomy. Why shouldn't you and your doctor decide what is in your best interests? Why shouldn't you have the option to choose your doctor?

Nevertheless, all players in the business of healthcare, such as government and commercial payers and funders, employers, hospitals, pharma, physicians, and consumers, are in agreement that our present system of healthcare delivery and funding is in need of repair and innovations. There is consensus that services and payment should be

---

29   John Kelley et al., "The Influence of the Patient-Clinician Relationship on Healthcare Outcomes: A Systematic Review and Meta-analysis of Randomized Controlled Trials," *PloS One* 9, no. 4 (April 9, 2014): e94207, https://doi.org/10.1371/journal.pone.0094207.

based on value, not volume. Value can be thought of as the quality of the service provided divided by the cost of the service. Thus, the higher quality of a given service provided at a fixed or equivalent cost will lead to increased value. But if increased cost is needed to increase quality, value will vary, depending on the relative level of quality and costs. This has led to proposals of various alternative payment models, some that are new and innovative, others that are variations on previous managed care approaches. Most models have introduced the concepts of shared risk and shared savings, whereby the healthcare provider will share the financial risk for poor outcomes as well as the financial rewards for optimized outcomes. In these newer models, preventive care becomes as important as the classical approaches of treating established disease.

Methods of achieving these lofty goals are presently being tested or developed. Alternative payment models include providing "capitated" predetermined payments for each patient over a period of time (per year, for example), something that has been done in modified form in years past by managed care organizations. Such an approach puts all the financial risk on the provider (physician, hospital systems, etc.) but incentivizes quality outcomes and judicious utilization of resources and eliminates administrative burdens such as preauthorizations. Less radical methods are to provide "global" payments for a diagnostic category or series of services, or payments for "episodes of care"; for example, a new epilepsy patient will have episodes of initial evaluation, diagnostic testing, and initial treatment and then additional episodes, depending on response to treatment or other needs based on the assessment and treatment algorithm.

Other approaches have included "bundled" payments rather than payments for each submitted CPT code, something that has also been done in the past and presently with diagnostic-related groups (DRG) payments, which primarily involve hospital systems. Some physician proprietors have found that direct payment models (DPMs)—in which insurance payers are not involved and the patient provides a direct payment for services, which is a modification of an older fee-for-service model—work well and allow tremendous cost savings in running a practice due to the elimination of interfacing with insurance bureaucracies, as well as providing increased practice freedoms. Similarly, there are "concierge" practices that charge a membership or similar type of fee, but usually still bill insurances.

Thus, there are many opportunities for innovation and disruption for newer models of healthcare delivery and payment for services for special needs populations that eschew standard fee-for-service models. In the end successful alternative payment models will be a win-win for all involved.

A BETTER SYSTEM FOR DELIVERING QUALITY, COST-EFFECTIVE CARE

What do we propose instead?

Our vision, in a nutshell, is to forgo the fee-for-service, cherry-picking reimbursement system and offer value-based care and bundled/global services within the framework of our patient- and family-centered Specialty Care Medical Home. Right now, every service line is reimbursed separately. Behavioral services have insurance- and government-mandated restrictions and hurdles like authorizations, denials, lack of complete coverage, and more. Medical services have similar but additional restraints and impediments. None of them are incentivized to work together, which is not simply more effective and efficient but also is the *only* way to produce consistently positive and optimized clinical outcomes that our patients deserve. Our vision brings these disciplines together, adding their areas of expertise synergistically, combining work in neurology, psychology, behavior therapy, creative arts therapy, and much more in an integrated, collaborative manner.

We propose a holistic, science-based model, the primary purpose of which is to promote optimized outcomes for the individuals and families who come to us in physical or emotional distress. Our relationship with them is unlike the transactional relationship of an insurance company or pharmaceutical company; it is deeply personal. We see their pain and go home each night thinking about what we might do to help them. They are *our* patients, *our* patients' families, people who came to us seeking relief and hoping we can provide it. They are not simply numbers on a spreadsheet. The highly skilled and caring practitioners in our practice entered their fields and studied for years in order to heal others in distress. We are personally inspired and motivated to treat and possibly cure sick people, to keep others healthy, to reduce their physical and emotional pain, to help them manage their conditions and enjoy the very best life possible.

For the neurologically fragile children, adolescents, and adults we treat, we have adopted a model that delivers optimized outcomes and cost-effective care in the long run. Our Specialty Care Medical Home® treats challenged and disabled individuals who require a clinical mindset that is willing to think outside the mainstream and utilize diagnostic protocols geared to better define and understand their issues. These individuals should be offered the latest diagnostic technologies and an array of standard and atypical treatment options that are personalized and precise: optimizing a treatment plan for the unique needs and diagnostic findings for an individual, rather than an average of group of similar people, as you have seen from some of the examples I have outlined.

All these services should be delivered within an integrated system of key clinicians from diverse but relevant fields of study and practice.

We feel that our approach to healthcare delivery for special needs populations is innovative and disruptive and is uniquely suited for implementing various proposed alternative payment models that have been discussed previously. We are confident that our ability to achieve optimized outcomes is applicable to shared risk and shared savings and accomplishes the goal of value-based care.

Part of the savings under such a system would be the simple disentanglement from insurance administration. If you think that sounds like hyperbole, consider this: research by Robert Kocher published in the *Harvard Business Review* found that for every six clinicians that a hospital or healthcare practice employs to deliver care, it must employ ten administrators to support them.[30] Most of those administrators handle insurance billing, collections, and compliance as a portion or the entirety of their jobs. In other words, only 37 percent of the people a patient encounters in a healthcare facility are actually providing the care that drew the patient there. That research is nine years old as of this writing. It is difficult to imagine that the ratio has done anything since then but tilt further toward more administrators.

It is conservatively estimated that one-third of healthcare costs in the United States are consumed by practice overhead and provider time spent billing.[31] Not one penny of that expenditure manifests in improved quality or more healthful outcomes.

The problem is not unique to healthcare facilities; families and the companies that employ them bear this burden as well. Research by Jeffrey Pepper and his team at Stanford University in 2019 found that the employees lose $21.6 billion a year spending time on the phone with health insurance companies, and employers lose another

---

30   Robert Kocher, "The Downside of Health Care Job Growth," *Harvard Business Review*, September 23, 2013, https://hbr.org/2013/09/the-downside-of-health-care-job-growth.

31   David Himmelstein et al., "Health Care Administrative Costs," *Annals of Internal Medicine* 172, no. 2 (2020): 134–142.

$26 billion a year from extra absence on the part of employees doing battle with health benefits administrators. Companies lose another $95 billion, the research estimates, from the reduced productivity that arises because people who spend time on the phone with health insurers are less satisfied with their jobs and seek alternative employment.[32]

Consider how this would have worked for Bobbi and her diagnostic odyssey in chapter 1. Correctly diagnosing her with a few simple, relatively inexpensive tests would have saved literally hundreds of thousands of dollars on nondiagnostic insurance-approved diagnostic tests, ineffective treatments, and avoidable hospitalizations.

> **Cheaper is not always less expensive; indeed, it often is not, especially when it comes to understanding patients as unique individuals with their individual health characteristics.**

More importantly, Bobbi lost more than a decade of her life to mistreatment that could have been avoided under a different healthcare delivery paradigm.

But cheaper is not always less expensive; indeed, it often is not, especially when it comes to understanding patients as unique individuals with their individual health characteristics. The investment in diagnostics on the front end for specialized care like ours is a cost-effective investment in delivering care that promises optimized outcomes. As the saying goes: "If you don't know where you're going, any road will get you there." We have found it makes economic as well as clinical sense to determine where we are going

---

32   Jeffrey Pfeffer et al., "Magnitude and Effects of 'Sludge' in Benefits Administration: How Health Insurance Hassles Burden Workers and Cost Employers," *Academy of Management Discoveries* 6 (2020): 325–340.

with each patient and to develop a customized treatment plan for them.

The current patchwork US healthcare system allocates an astronomical number of dollars—3.6 trillion of them in 2018, to be exact—for thousands of services whose value is … well, no one precisely knows. Our nation ranks forty-sixth in the world in life expectancy, behind Qatar, Poland, Lebanon, Cuba, and Estonia. If the ultimate measure of a healthcare system is the longevity of its users, that is not an especially auspicious indicator. (I am not advocating for longevity as the comprehensive metric for healthcare value; after all, individuals are responsible for a host of decisions that affect their longevity and on which the healthcare system cannot exert any influence.

> **Our nation ranks forty-sixth in the world in life expectancy, behind Qatar, Poland, Lebanon, Cuba, and Estonia. If the ultimate measure of a healthcare system is the longevity of its users, that is not an especially auspicious indicator.**

However, there is intuitively some correlation between the two.) More to the point, without a robust structure of outcome measurement for integrated systems of care, it is impossible to ascertain its cost-effectiveness.

As I've noted, measuring the outcomes of individual units of activity does little to represent the efficacy of an integrated system of care. Fortunately, the insurance industry's gravitation toward big data is beginning to reveal the true value of a collaborative and cohesive model, like the one we execute and advocate. At the same time, insurance continues to reimburse for care that produces no results but follows the formula of prescribed services and activities. The systemic result is that it costs $2 million to treat a child with autism through adolescence, irrespective of the degree of improvement in behavior, and then funding stops for important services as an adult, often leading to loss of previous gains: not a very cost-effective approach over the long run.[33]

The value of a unified model of care delivery is very personal to Karen, whose son Connor was disruptive from the age of two. Even in daycare, Connor was coming home with incident reports building the case for his removal from the program.

"It was so hard to love him through it," she told us. "Every day we were getting negativity from daycares and teachers and other parents. Everybody just wants us to fix it, wants us to control our wild child. We were taking all of the appropriate steps, but no one could give us an answer, definitively, as to what was wrong with our son."

The reason, as you could probably have predicted by now, is that Connor's treatment was based on a faulty diagnosis and executed by individual practitioners working, if not quite in silos, then without sufficient communication or collaboration. Our practice ordered tests that had never been considered before. Our developmental pediatrician and neuropsychologist evaluated the results with Connor's parents and determined that he had an underlying neurobiological disorder manifesting with symptoms and signs of autism spectrum disorder, disruptive mood dysregulation disorder, and ADHD. We offered Karen and Connor's father two pages of recommendations for his treatment that were customized to his suite of conditions.

"So after five years of basically beating our heads against the wall, we were given a report that was a how-to manual for our son,"

---

33   Ariane Buescher et al., "Costs of Autism Spectrum Disorders in the United Kingdom and the United States," *Journal of the American Medical Association Pediatrics* 168 (2014): 721–728, doi: 10.1001/jamapediatrics.2014.210.

she said. Karen reported that the family was able to take an enjoyable vacation to Disney World, something unthinkable during Connor's first seven years. That is a long way from struggling to love their challenging child.

Everyone's talking about outcomes, and certainly that's what you want if you are dealing with any of the issues we treat. But there is not just one kind of outcome, as I have suggested, because the outcome of a single, fragmented unit of activity by a single practitioner is not the same as the outcome of a coordinated portfolio of care delivered by a team of clinicians synergistically. We are going to explore that and more in the next chapter.

CHAPTER 4

Producing
Optimized Outcomes

A missing piece of pediatric autism services specifically and neurological assessment and treatment generally is the question of what successful outcomes look like. This lends itself to highly variable answers, depending on the child, their condition, and its severity, and it often comes with inconsistencies. That is, we can often only speculate what clinical success might look like. For parents who bring in a child at the severe end of the autism spectrum, success may be defined by very modest gains in basic life skills. They might never acquire language, build relationships, or live independently but can nonetheless enjoy a higher quality of life. Treatment of a child at the other end of the spectrum might aim for complete independence and functional life skills.

Defining optimized outcomes requires defining optimized objectives and developing relevant measures for successful results. This is harder than it sounds; clinicians often are unable to devote the time and effort this requires. After all, this process establishes the starting and ending points and the process by which it is determined that the desired clinical outcome has been achieved.

Which brings us to Matt's story.

Matt came to us at the age of six, having spent five of those years in the grip of an incapacitating and demoralizing condition—cyclical vomiting syndrome. Roughly every ninety days since he was a year old, Matt would experience excruciating "ice-pick" headaches, so called because they feel as if an ice pick is being jabbed into the victim's temples. Nausea, dizziness, light sensitivity, and abdominal pain would disable him for about a week before the vomiting would begin, hours and hours of vomiting lasting a day or two, with the added risk of dehydration to complicate an already dire situation. The other symptoms would persist for another week after that, keeping Matt out of school for three weeks every three months—like clockwork. Nothing in particular seemed to trigger Matt's vomiting except the calendar, and there didn't seem to be much his doctors could do.

Cyclical vomiting syndrome (CVS) is not well understood, and the typical treatment of antinausea/antiemetic (antivomiting) drugs, like ondansetron (Zofran) and promethazine (Phenergan); antivertigo drugs, like meclizine (Antivert); and antianxiety drugs, like lorazepam (Ativan), has a spotty track record. Often clinicians seek the triggers—like certain foods, excitement, anxiety, or physical exhaustion—and help patients learn how to avoid or manage them. None of this had worked for Matt. His family had begun accepting the fact that this was his fate for the foreseeable future.

We can all commiserate with the discomfort and pain involved in this condition, but consider how utterly debilitating it had to be for Matt and his parents. For seventy days the family could enjoy the calm, laden with dread of what was to come. Then, predictably, family life was turned upside down, and Matt's parents had to watch their child suffer for three weeks, punctuated by two days of abject misery.

Imagine watching your five-year-old endure this literally every three months, as predictable as the change of seasons.

Exacerbating the horror for Matt's mother was guilt—and not just the usual maternal guilt connected with watching her little boy suffer. An epileptic herself, she was tortured with the fear that the medications she took for her condition while pregnant with Matt had caused his condition. The whole situation, which I haven't even fully described, would lead any reasonable person to despair.

Six years passed without any improvement in Matt's condition, and the family sought out an additional opinion from NeurAbilities. They were hopeful our integrated, multidisciplinary, holistic, and comprehensive clinical model would be able to provide them solutions to Matt's dilemma. And we embraced the challenge.

One of several distinguishing features of our organization is the inclusion of medical genetics and the utilization of cutting-edge genetic testing. Dr. Richard Boles, a medical geneticist, pediatrician, and director of our NeuroGenomics program, brings decades of clinical and research experience at major academic centers, along with experience in pioneering biotechnology and genomics laboratories. Part of our secret sauce, Dr. Boles's skills and insights provide an essential diagnostic component and perspective to cases that patients rarely experience anywhere else.

In the case of Matt, we recognized that his disorder might have a genetic or other biological cause and engaged in a comprehensive assessment of his condition. As I've previously mentioned, we invest time and effort in diagnostics that may find individual differences to unlock a path for a better outcome. For Matt, this included genetic testing that revealed a genetic variation that causes a problem in how calcium enters and exits cells in his brain, a condition known as (calcium) channelopathy.

We administered to Matt an old and simple medication that can temper the influx of calcium and decrease excitability of the brain cells affected. The drug, acetazolamide, is a diuretic, more often used to treat the buildup of fluid in conditions like glaucoma and congestive heart failure or to lower blood pressure. Paradoxically, its potential adverse effects include fatigue, nausea, vomiting, abdominal pain, and diarrhea—the very conditions we were treating in Matt. Employing our "Start low and go slow" philosophy for medication titration, where we attempt to administer the lowest dose that provides beneficial effects (or "minimally effective dose"), we eased Matt onto acetazolamide, and over the course of the year, his symptoms slowly resolved, to the point that a year later he was totally symptom free. Matt is ten now, and his condition is completely under control with this simple and easily tolerated medication. He can go to school without interruption, his mother is free to work outside the home, family life is back to normal, and Matt's quality of life is immeasurably improved. Matt's mother told us we had "saved his life."

I tell you this story because it is the holy grail of medical practice. A patient with a debilitating condition walked through our doors and achieved total remediation simply, inexpensively, and completely. I don't say he is "cured" because he still has the condition and the genetic variant; it is just under control for now. His quality of life is discernibly and dramatically improved in what appears to be a sustainable way. For Matt, the approach of personalized and precision medicine informed our treatment interventions that increased potential efficacy. When examining efficacy "statistics" for treatment interventions, a clinical study may show a statistically significant benefit of, say, improvement in 60 percent of patients, but for the individual, the treatment either works or does not, or is 0 percent or 100 percent effective. Or a clinical research study for an antiepileptic drug for suppressing seizures in those with severe, intractable epilepsy may show a reduction of daily seizures from one hundred to fifty, which is statistically significant (and may be sufficient to obtain regulatory approval for general use) but is not necessarily clinically relevant, as fifty seizures a day is still very debilitating. Identifying and measuring outcomes is the subject of much debate in our industry. Clinical outcome measures determine whether we have achieved our goal for each of our patients. But how best to measure outcomes that are not just statistically significant but clinically relevant?

And that is the point of this chapter.

Outcome measures are used to assess whether a clinical objective has been achieved. But not all objectives—and therefore not all outcomes—are equally meaningful. Indeed, there is no defined baseline in clinical use against which to measure progress in the behavioral field. Common sense suggests employing behavioral reductionism—reducing the incidence of problematic behaviors—but there are limits to it use. For negative behaviors we seek to limit, for example, if our objective is to reduce self-injurious behavior, we define the behavior in question and measure its frequency and intensity. A child who hits himself repeatedly might be observed during and after treatment to determine whether he hit himself less often (e.g., five times in an hour rather than ten). Including an intensity measure—admittedly more subjective—provides a more nuanced and accurate picture. In the same example, we might document whether the blows to his head involved a fist or open hand, whether they were glancing blows or direct hits to hard structures like the skull or soft targets like the eyes.

All of this helps clinicians to fashion a treatment plan that might involve ignoring (i.e., not rewarding with attention) the behavior, correcting it, distracting or redirecting the child, reinforcing noninjurious

behavior, or even something as blunt as protecting the child from the inevitable hitting with a helmet or other shield. Developing these outcomes
is more a process of trial and error, adoption of commonly accepted best
practices, and even inertia (i.e., doing what has always been done) than
the use of a rigorous set of guidelines within the relevant professions.

The *Diagnostic and Statistical Manual of Mental Disorders, Fifth
Edition*, commonly known as the DSM-5, is the taxonomic and diagnostic tool produced by the American Psychiatric Association, serving
as the principal authority for psychiatric diagnoses. But certain maladaptive behaviors elude classification as a disorder. DSM-5 classifies
behavior types, like nonsuicidal self-injury, as symptoms of other conditions, like bipolar disorder, and not as separate, stand-alone disorders.
In this particular case, its authors determined that additional empirical
data was necessary before classifying nonsuicidal self-injury as a disorder.
Consequently, outcome measurements of behaviors with a neurological
etiology are not systematically addressed in DSM-5, leaving clinicians
to rely on tried-and-true treatments that might vary from practice to
practice. Furthermore, the DSM-5 does not account for medical or
biological causes of self-injurious behaviors, or for most of the diagnoses
in the DSM-5, as a DSM-5 diagnosis can often be assigned regardless
of the biological causes or contributions. Conversely, behavioral data
can be highly informative for clinical management, regardless of the
DSM-5 diagnosis or classification.

Creating and utilizing reliable and objective outcome measures
for various neurological and neurodevelopmental disorders and disabilities can also be problematic. Often outcomes are based on subjective "impressions" of the patient, clinician, or other observer as to
whether someone is doing the same, better, or worse compared to a
previous time point. And although such impressions can be quantified
using numerical scales, the results can be somewhat influenced by

bias, lack of standardization, and other factors. Neuropsychological testing provides empirical, quantified, normative, and reliable data on cognitive function and thus can be utilized as an important outcome measure for clinical use or research studies, but it is labor intensive, and many measures are not repeatable within a year. Neurophysiological data is important objective information, such as HD-EEG demonstrating suppression of abnormal electrical discharges after a therapeutic intervention, especially if correlating to improved cognitive and behavioral functioning. There are computerized tests that can quantify responses correlating to attention and vigilance.

Academic productivity can provide outcome information. Maintaining headache or sleep diaries provides inputs concerning frequency, intensity, and disruption to life activities but can also be influenced by bias and lack of standardization. And a host of laboratory tests may add to objective outcome data. Overall, there are an array of subjective and objective measures that can contribute to determining the benefit or efficacy of a treatment intervention, but can have intrinsic constraints or limits, particularly for certain neurodevelopmental/neuropsychiatric diagnoses, and may not necessarily translate to clinical relevance and quality of life.

WILL MY CHILD BE TYPICAL?

What then, for example, is a good outcome for a child with autism spectrum disorder? This is an issue with which clinicians in the field struggle every day, particularly when discussing the prognosis with parents. Treatment for ASD is a lifelong effort; requires a team of caring people, including parents, other family members, teachers, physicians, behaviorists, and others; and is uncertain from the start. The earlier treatment can begin in a child's life, the better the outcomes, adding another variable into the mix.

Moreover, ASD is rarely a stand-alone condition. People with autism face increased risk for a litany of comorbidities, including physical health issues like obesity, gastrointestinal and immune function issues, metabolic and sleep disorders, and epilepsy; of psychological and emotional issues, including anxiety, depression, and ADHD; and of behavioral issues in adolescence and adulthood, including substance abuse, legal problems, and increased risk of being bullied.

The ultimate outcome in which a child "recovers" and grows up to be indistinguishable from neurotypical adults is somewhere between uncommon and rare. As I previously shared earlier in the book, we don't refer to these children as "cured" for a couple of reasons. First, a neurotypical perspective of how we conduct ourselves is simply the norm, not an objective right or wrong. We deal with a neuro-diverse universe where every individual brain functions differently. High-functioning individuals with autism can engage in perfectly functional relationships with each other, defined by autistic norms in which neurotypical individuals would appear to be ill adapted. The neurotypical use of eye contact when engaging with others may cause increased anxiety for a high-functioning person with autism. Second, and more to the point, individuals with autism—that is, whose brains are wired differently—do not stop having autism. Their brains do not necessarily become rewired, although a subset experiences a degree of brain reorganization over time due to brain plasticity; they simply learn how to manage in a neurotypical world. Research has found that somewhere between 3 percent and 25 percent of individuals diagnosed with ASD as children no longer meet the criteria for the diagnosis as adults.[34] The unacceptably wide range of these findings

---

34 Deborah Anderson, "Predicting Young Adult Outcome among More and Less Cogni-
    tively Able Individuals with Autism Spectrum Disorders," *Journal of Child Psychology
    and Psychiatry, and Allied Disciplines* 55, no. 5 (2014): 485–494, doi:10.1111/jcpp.12178.

is the result of multiple studies employing varied methodology and sample sets and questions about subjective diagnostic measures, both in childhood and adulthood.

With that said, researchers and clinicians have identified a variety of predictors of positive outcomes that can help clinicians offer parents a clearer picture of the upper and lower limits of their children's prognosis. These predictors include IQ, ability to process language, verbal and motor imitation, fine motor control, and the age of intervention. An early ability to understand and communicate through language is a good early predictor of future success in treatment. This highlights the importance of early diagnosis and treatment to help the child progress by such a young age. Even knowing that, the range of outcomes is quite large and affected by these other factors and more.

> Our nation struggles to confront an epidemic of autism that is now estimated to affect one in every thirty-six children born in 2018.

Research has found that the attitudes and behaviors of parents and other stakeholders also affect the long-term prognosis of children with autism. Barriers to success include a poor person-environment fit, stakeholder issues with their proper role, and a lack of community services. A poor person-environment fit might involve placing a young adult with greater potential in a limiting workplace role that stunts their achievement. An example of stakeholder issues would be parents or others involved in a child's life doing things for them that they could learn to do for themselves. In addition, a lack of community services is an endemic problem facing almost all children with autism, as our nation struggles to confront an epidemic of autism that is now estimated to affect one in every thirty-six children aged eight years in 2020.[35]

A host of other factors can affect the reduction in maladaptive behaviors and increase adults' ability to perform activities of daily living. Positive soft-skill variables would not surprise you: they include greater-quality parent-child relationships and greater assimilation in academic and social activities in school.

Taken together, the collection of ingredients traversing time—behavioral and medical treatment, home life, school and community support, the quality of relationships, and the child's starting point—all conspire to form the broad outline of their potential. But predicting the ultimate treatment trajectory and outcome of a two-year-old with any kind of definitive certainty is fraught with inaccuracies. That said, parents do want answers.

CURE VERSUS TREATMENT

When I refer to autism as not having a "cure" in a classical way, I am reminded of my early days in medical residency during the height of the AIDS crisis. Until the COVID-19 pandemic hit, it was difficult for people who didn't live through those early years of the AIDS pandemic to understand the fear and pain AIDS caused. Indeed, in the early years of the AIDS pandemic, it was even worse than COVID-19 in several very important ways: (1) the modes of transmission and infection were not well understood, (2) AIDS caused severe disease in all affected children and adults, usually resulting in death, and (3) there were no cures and very few effective treatments. Before we identified the virus that caused AIDS—the human immunodeficiency virus, or HIV—and even for a few years after we did, AIDS killed the majority of people

---

35   Maenner, "Prevalence and Characteristics of Autism Spectrum Disorder Among Children Aged 8 Years," 2023.

who contracted it, and before it did, it ravaged their bodies in terrible ways. AIDS demoralizes and dehumanizes before it kills, and initially it was noted that it spread like wildfire among specific populations, most notably, but not exclusively, young gay men. AIDS was rampant at a time when being gay already carried a heavy social stigma, complicating the effort to stem its spread. Shortly thereafter, it became clear that HIV/AIDS was not restricted to the gay community but was rampant among intravenous drug users, those who received tainted blood transfusions, and babies born to HIV-infected mothers. Even heterosexuals were susceptible via unprotected sex.

Eventually, though, we developed the tools to fight the virus to a draw. There remains today no effective vaccine for HIV, but we can control its spread through behavioral changes and prophylactic measures; prevent many of the opportunistic, deadly infections that it causes with judicious use of antimicrobials; and reduce HIV viral loads to the level of undetectability using antiretroviral drugs. In the 1980s, people died of AIDS; today they live with HIV. Those early clinical lessons have guided me throughout my medical career.

Autism is not a fatal condition, but it has similarities in the sense that it is endemic and chronic and can improve with early and ongoing treatments and therapies. As I mentioned, we cannot cure autism, and even if we could, many in the

Many individuals with autism are distinguishable from other adults but can take care of themselves, communicate effectively, have fulfilling relationships, display creativity, and be professionally successful.

autistic community would object, at least to curing high-functioning individuals who can enjoy quality, independent lives but whose perspective is different from neurotypical individuals. Many individuals with autism are distinguishable from other adults but can take care of themselves, communicate effectively, have fulfilling relationships, display creativity, and be professionally successful.

Luke is a good example of how we can achieve positive outcomes that are a long way from a cure. A young man in his twenties with severe autism but the very powerful advantage of hypervigilant and loving parents, Luke was our patient for years. His parents were relentless in their quest to provide their son with the best life possible given his condition, the kinds of partners who invigorate and motivate the professionals in our practice. While we provided a host of integrated services to Luke several times a week for more than a decade, his parents took the initiative to create a community center where young autistic adults could gather with like-minded individuals for social activities and friendships. At Luke's Place, located in Audubon, New Jersey, the members attend dances, go on field trips, enjoy communal meals, and experience all the social activities one associates with a community center.

Luke is not "cured"—far from it. He has severe autism and challenges in his life. He is not fully independent and probably never will be. But he has the supports he needs, has learned to communicate and function well within the parameters of his supportive environment, and perhaps, in the ultimate evidence of his improved function, hasn't needed our services for years. And through Luke's Place, he and his family have helped so many others with similar challenges. I believe everyone involved in Luke's care fifteen years ago would have agreed that this is a very auspicious outcome, given Luke's condition when we first began seeing him. This positive outcome was made possible by many individuals and entities—first and foremost his parents; other family members who provided support; the many therapists, behaviorists, and physicians who worked with him in and outside of our organization; teachers and other educators who collaborated with us; and many, many other individuals who comprised his care-support team.

WHAT IS THE *SPECTRUM* IN AUTISM SPECTRUM DISORDERS?

Not all children are the same. Autism has a spectrum for a reason—because there is a rainbow of shades, hues, gradients, and intensities of autism that are unique to each child with the condition. Some children, regardless of the length, intensity, and professionalism of their treatment, will never gain the ability to talk. Other individuals become performers with just a few coping tools before they light out on their own. As advocates often say, when you've met one person with autism, you've met one person with autism. At some point, we must define what we mean by outcomes.

Let's start this discussion by examining the spectrum. Individuals with autism are as different from each other as you and me. I have curly hair, love opera, and am generally stoic—even in the face of adversity or grief. (It is important to be clear that stoic people don't *feel* the heartbreak less; we are merely reticent to display those feelings, particularly in an overly demonstrative way.)

> **Autism has a spectrum for a reason—because there is a rainbow of shades, hues, gradients, and intensities of autism that are unique to each child with the condition.**

The odds are quite good that you do not share all three of these characteristics, and if you do, we can pick three others on which we diverge. The same is true for children with autism, even within their diagnosis. They vary in their ability to communicate; the number and intensity of their physical, psychological, and behavioral comorbidities; their ability to grasp social cues; their intellectual ability; and so on, and in the extant conditions surrounding them, like the coping abilities of their parents. Although we clinicians must form a diagnosis very early on in our relationship with a patient, we really cannot pinpoint where "on the spectrum" a child is until after many hours of observation and investigation.

The diagnosis of autism has been affected by the "lumpers" versus "splitters" approaches of psychiatry and neurology. Historically, there has been a philosophical split between the two disciplines, with psychiatrists tending to define a group of symptoms such as repetitive behaviors, social impairments, poor eye contact, and communication or language deficits and "lump" them into one diagnosis: "autistic disorder." But as we have discussed, the neurobiological approach to autism is to be diagnosis agnostic and "split" this group with similar symptoms and divide them into clinical or biological subgroups, depending on various criteria and neurodiagnostic findings. Although the broad, general diagnosis of autism is useful for categorizing children for receiving educational interventions, behavioral therapies, and more, the latter "splitting" approach is more neurologically relevant and necessary for precision medicine. In the DSM editions prior to the release of DSM-5, there was the umbrella diagnosis of "pervasive developmental disorders" (PDD), and underneath this umbrella five subtypes (autistic disorder, PDD-not otherwise specified, Asperger disorder or Asperger syndrome, Rett disorder, and childhood disintegrative disorder)—all diagnoses that could be assigned, regardless of biological causes or contributions.

Since the features of the subtypes were based on behavioral and developmental observations, there often were much confusion and many inaccuracies in diagnosis, leading to a lack of individualized therapies. The latest edition of the DSM released in 2013 (DSM-5) continued this "lumping" philosophy and replaced the PDD umbrella and its subtypes with one diagnostic term, *autistic disorder*, which is commonly referred to as autism spectrum disorder (ASD). Rather than apply behavioral subtypes, as was done under the PDD umbrella, the DSM-5 classifies three severity levels and asks whether there is accompanying intellectual impairment, language impairment, or catatonia; associations with other neurodevelopmental, mental, or behavioral disorders; or known medical or genetic conditions or other contributing environmental factors.

DSM-5 also included a new diagnosis called social pragmatic communication disorder, with many of the communication impairments seen in ASD but without other significant features of ASD. The change in the psychiatric diagnosis of ASD caused some consternation among some neurodiversity groups, such as those with Asperger disorder, who tend to be highly intelligent and "high functioning" with milder symptoms of autism. The Asperger diagnosis was eliminated in the DSM-5, although some of these individuals may qualify for social pragmatic communication disorder or other psychiatric diagnoses, or if they already have an established Asperger diagnosis, they can be assigned autism spectrum disorder. Likewise, you may have heard the term "high-functioning autism," but it is not a diagnosis in the DSM-5 and was never an official psychiatric diagnosis. Other former PDD subtypes, such as Rett syndrome, which was discovered to have a genetic mutation in the MECP gene, again illustrate the many neurobiological causes of autism.

Under the DSM-5, the criteria for a diagnosis of autism spectrum disorder are now a dyad of two broad categories of deficits in (1) social communication and interaction, and (2) restricted, repetitive behavior patterns, both of varying degrees and severities. As defined by the DSM-5:

DSM-5 AUTISM DIAGNOSTIC CRITERIA

A. **Persistent deficits in social communication and social interaction across multiple contexts, as manifested by the following, currently or by history (examples are illustrative, not exhaustive, see text):**

   1. Deficits in social-emotional reciprocity, ranging, for example, from abnormal social approach and failure of normal back-and-forth conversation; to reduced sharing of interests, emotions, or affect; to failure to initiate or respond to social interactions.

   2. Deficits in nonverbal communicative behaviors used for social interaction, ranging, for example, from poorly integrated verbal and nonverbal communication; to abnormalities in eye contact and body language or deficits in understanding and use of gestures; to a total lack of facial expressions and nonverbal communication.

   3. Deficits in developing, maintaining, and understanding relationships, ranging, for example, from difficulties adjusting behavior to suit various social contexts; to difficulties in sharing imaginative play or in making friends; to absence of interest in peers.

Specify current severity: severity is based on social communication impairments and restricted repetitive patterns of behavior. (See below.)

B. **Restricted, repetitive patterns of behavior, interests, or activities, as manifested by at least two of the following, currently or by history (examples are illustrative, not exhaustive; see text):**

   1. Stereotyped or repetitive motor movements, use of objects, or speech (e.g., simple motor stereotypies, lining up toys or flipping objects, echolalia, idiosyncratic phrases).

2. Insistence on sameness, inflexible adherence to routines, or ritualized patterns or verbal nonverbal behavior (e.g., extreme distress at small changes, difficulties with transitions, rigid thinking patterns, greeting rituals, need to take same route or eat food every day).

3. Highly restricted, fixated interests that are abnormal in intensity or focus (e.g., strong attachment to or preoccupation with unusual objects, excessively circumscribed or perseverative interest).

4. Hyper- or hyporeactivity to sensory input or unusual interests in sensory aspects of the environment (e.g., apparent indifference to pain/temperature, adverse response to specific sounds or textures, excessive smelling or touching of objects, visual fascination with lights or movement).

Specify current severity: Severity is based on social communication impairments and restricted, repetitive patterns of behavior. (See below.)

C. Symptoms must be present in the early developmental period (but may not become fully manifest until social demands exceed limited capacities or may be masked by learned strategies in later life).

D. Symptoms cause clinically significant impairment in social, occupational, or other important areas of current functioning.

E. These disturbances are not better explained by intellectual disability (intellectual developmental disorder) or global developmental delay. Intellectual disability and autism spectrum disorder frequently co-occur; to make comorbid diagnoses of autism spectrum disorder and intellectual disability, social communication should be below that expected for general developmental level.

Note: Individuals with a well-established DSM-IV diagnosis of autistic disorder, Asperger disorder, or pervasive developmental disorder not otherwise specified should be given the diagnosis of autism spectrum disorder. Individuals who have marked deficits in social communication, but whose symptoms do not otherwise meet criteria for autism spectrum disorder, should be evaluated for social (pragmatic) communication disorder.

Note: A diagnosis of Autism Spectrum Disorder is met if criteria A-E are satisfied.

Specify if:

❏ **With or without accompanying intellectual impairment**

❏ **With or without accompanying language impairment**

❏ **Associated with another neurodevelopmental, mental, or behavioral disorder**

❏ **With catatonia**

❏ **Associated with a known medical or genetic condition or environmental factor**

TABLE: SEVERITY LEVELS FOR AUTISM SPECTRUM DISORDER

SEVERITY LEVEL	SOCIAL COMMUNICATION	RESTRICTED, REPETITIVE BEHAVIORS
Level 3 "Requiring very substantial support"	Severe deficits in verbal and nonverbal social communication skills cause severe impairments in functioning, very limited initiation of social interactions, and minimal response to social overtures from others. For example, a person with few words of intelligible speech who rarely initiates interaction and, when he or she does, makes unusual approaches to meet needs only and responds to only very direct social approaches.	Inflexibility of behavior, extreme difficulty coping with change, or other restricted/repetitive behaviors markedly interfere with functioning in all spheres. Great distress/difficulty changing focus or action.
Level 2 "Requiring substantial support"	Marked deficits in verbal and nonverbal social communication skills, social impairments apparent even with supports in place, limited initiation of social interactions, and reduced or abnormal responses to social overtures from others. For example, a person who speaks simple sentences, whose interaction is limited to narrow special interests, and has markedly odd nonverbal communication.	Inflexibility of behavior, difficulty coping with change, or other restricted/repetitive behaviors appear frequently enough to be obvious to the casual observer and interfere with functioning in a variety of contexts. Distress and/or difficulty changing focus or action.

Level 1 "Requiring support"	Without supports in place, deficits in social communication cause noticeable impairments. Difficulty initiating social interactions, and clear examples of atypical or unsuccessful response to social overtures of others. May appear to have decreased interest in social interactions. For example, a person who is able to speak in full sentences and engages in communication but whose to-and-fro conversation with others fails and whose attempts to make friends are odd and typically unsuccessful.	Inflexibility of behavior causes significant interference with functioning in one or more contexts. Difficulty switching between activities. Problems of organization and planning hamper independence.

Diagnostic and Statistical Manual of Mental Disorders Fifth Edition,
American Psychiatric Association, 2013

But as I have emphasized throughout, for our clinical model, where we are diagnosis agnostic, we are not as concerned about the nonspecific diagnosis of ASD but rather the underlying clinical profile and biological phenotype. We approach our patients as individuals so that we can personalize their treatment. It is worth repeating Dr. Frazier's admonition of the DSM-5 criteria for ASD that "neurobiological studies will be useful for determining ... whether the DSM-5 ASD diagnosis can be empirically parsed into biologically meaningful subphenotypes."

The abilities of individuals with autism spectrum disorder to learn, process information, and socialize cover the full range from savant to severely curtailed. Some will live independent, successful lives, and others will struggle with the activities of daily living their entire existence. Eminent individuals in the arts, science, and business confirmed or believed to be somewhere on the autism spectrum, albeit mostly "high functioning," include Albert Einstein, Bill Gates, Anthony Hopkins, Isaac Newton, Bobby Fischer, Stanley Kubrick, Satoshi Tajiri (creator of Pokémon), the animal scientist Dr. Temple Grandin, and Mozart. Many individuals with lower-functioning ASD associated with other physical or neurological handicaps displayed amazing "savant" talents, like Kim "Rain Man" Peek, the nineteenth-century master pianist "Blind" Tom Wiggins, the sculptor Alonzo Clemons, and many, many more.

When a child enters our practice, or any autism practice, they are presenting with some or all of these symptoms and even others I have not articulated. Once we have assessed the person, performed appropriate neurodiagnostic testing, and determined a diagnosis, we devise a treatment plan customized to addressing the conditions and behaviors that are preventing them from having a higher quality of life. As I've mentioned, we don't treat autism as a single entity but rather we target the underlying mechanisms, causes, and contributions to various symptoms and clinical manifestations of each individual. Obviously, children with ASD will present many of the same issues, and consequently some of their treatment plans will look similar, with overlapping interventions and therapies. But it is rare that any two therapeutic regimens are exactly alike because no two patients are exactly alike.

This process is not unique to our work: physicians generally will assess, diagnose, and develop a treatment plan. Most treatment plans include goals that have measurable objective and subjective outcomes; that is, we must be able to test whether we have achieved our long- and short-term goals in order to evaluate the efficacy of our treatment. The development of these outcomes, particularly short-term metrics that guide our daily work, is a combination of art and science and includes use of tools created out of the best practice standards in each field.

Consider this example: our long-term goal for a child with moderate ASD might be to help them gain language skills, navigate social situations, and live with some level of independence. We would develop short-term outcomes for our work with that child, designed to lead iteratively over time to those long-term goals. Examples of this include positive change in adaptive (daily living) skills and reduction in negative behaviors. Specifically, with respect to behavior management, we might seek to reduce the frequency and intensity of a child hitting himself or reduce the number of violent outbursts when confronted with a particular stimulus. With that as an objective, we can fashion a specific set of therapeutic actions to address the issues in question. This is another way we are treating the unique individual and not his or her diagnosis. Over time, our goal would be to eliminate this behavior completely. For adaptive behaviors, we might establish a short-term goal of pointing to something that a child cannot verbalize or repeating a question he has heard to unlock a situation. In so doing, children build skills that can help them transition into adulthood with the ability to navigate daily life in a neurotypical world.

NOT JUST OUTCOMES—OPTIMIZED OUTCOMES

As clinical research on autism and other neurological disorders advances, we are confronting a new issue in measuring outcomes: the difference between statistically significant outcomes and optimized ones. Previously I provided the example of severe epilepsy, in which a new drug may be found that reduce seizures from one hundred to fifty per day. That drug will get approved by the FDA because its impact is immense and statistically significant—cutting seizures by 50 percent. In a vacuum, a 50 percent reduction in seizure frequency is an outstanding result. But humans don't live in a vacuum; we live real lives that cannot merely be described by sterile data. If somebody is still having fifty seizures a day, their life has not changed very much. Whether a patient has four seizures every hour or two seizures every hour, they still can't work, drive a car, ride a bicycle, socialize, build relationships, or even leave the house for the most part. A pharmaceutical company that has spent millions of dollars developing an anti-epileptic medication and validating it through double-blind studies and massive documentation of efficacy will get FDA approval for marketing its new product, even though its use may have minimal practical impact.

Another example is the new Alzheimer's drug, aducanumab (Aduhelm): the first new drug for this insidious disease in twenty years. This very expensive drug was approved by the Food and Drug Administration (FDA) as it was shown to reduce the burden of beta-amyloid protein in the brain (a protein hypothesized to be a pathological mechanism for developing Alzheimer's). Yet results were uncertain in terms of the clinical benefit of slowing cognitive decline. The FDA's own independent advisory panel of experts and consultants recommended against approving the drug based on equivocal clinical outcomes, but the FDA approved this very expensive drug anyway. The FDA did require the makers of aducanumab to do additional studies of clinical benefit, but this created additional controversy, as there would be little incentive for patients to enroll in such studies if the drug were already available by prescription.

This is the tension between statistical significance and clinical relevance, and it fails to account for all the externalities. Every drug has side effects, creating a whole new trade-off between the therapeutic clinical gains the drug produces and its malign side effects. When utilizing pharmacological interventions for autism, we regularly choose from a menu of options that includes pharmaceuticals that regulate negative behaviors but have the potential for creating paradoxical adverse behaviors. It requires us to balance efficacy against toxicity and benefit versus risk and also account for affordability.

For example, the drug risperidone is commonly prescribed as an antipsychotic for schizophrenia and for the adverse behaviors of autism. The list of common behavioral and physical side effects runs to twenty-one items, including aggressive behavior, anxiety, difficulty speaking or swallowing, loss of balance, memory problems, muscle spasms, skin rash, trembling hands, trouble sleeping, and blurred vision. Most concerning is the ability to induce tardive dyskinesia, which is an uncontrolled movement disorder that may not necessarily resolve. Risperidone can be a very useful drug in select cases, whereby the benefits outweigh the risks, but in other cases the risk-to-benefit calculus is not favorable. Clinicians always bear in mind the tenets of "Do no harm" and "The cure should not be more harmful than the disease"—you would not want to burn down your house to kill a mosquito.

Using risperidone, it is possible to achieve the optimized outcome of reducing the symptoms of schizophrenia or maladaptive behaviors of autism. But in some cases, adverse side effects such as constant trembling, involuntary movements, memory loss, or paradoxical aggressiveness will limit or obviate its use. These types of dilemmas are a common part of providing pragmatic clinical management of patients receiving potent and potentially dangerous medications.

Thus, any treatment, but especially pharmacological and biological treatments, needs to be respected and used thoughtfully and pragmatically. In our clinical model, we consider the full matrix of outcomes in a systematic way, guided by a philosophy that focuses on the whole patient and their specific needs. First, we always attempt to optimize nonpharmacological treatments. Prescribing a pill is simple; therapeutic interventions take time and effort. Behavioral therapy rarely has a side effect profile and generally does not wear off when the patient ends treatment. Behavioral therapy provides a patient or his or her family with a set of tools to manage their behavior and develop coping skills, which are generalizable and can be sustainable. When possible, we prefer to invest the time and effort in helping patients become more functional through the utilization of nonpharmacological therapies rather than rely on medicine.

However, there are those individuals who will not achieve optimized outcomes without the use of adjunctive medications. When drugs comprise a reasonable option as part of a therapeutic regimen, we initially target medications offering the best combination of benefits with minimal risk of toxicity. I recognize that seems like common sense, but operationalizing it is more difficult and probably

> **When possible, we prefer to invest the time and effort in helping patients become more functional through the utilization of nonpharmacological therapies rather than rely on medicine.**

more uncommon than you imagine. It requires a concerted effort to review and analyze the matrix of benefits and detriments and apply them to each individual based on their specific circumstances. Pharmacogenomic information may also aid in identifying those drugs having a higher side effect risk or lower efficacy for the individual's unique pharmacogenetic profile. Additional baseline testing to eliminate other potential risks of medication toxicity, such as electrocardiograms or laboratory tests, may be indicated. This takes time and forethought that not every practice is prepared to dedicate. The more problematic and critical the clinical situation and the greater the benefits a particular medication may offer, the more potential toxic side effects we might be willing to tolerate.

We take that a step further with the "Start low; go slow" methodology of titrating medications in which we seek the minimally effective dose and monitor for side effects—either clinically observable, like behavior changes, or measurable through a blood test, like metabolic changes. We reject the notion that if a little bit of medicine is good, a lot must be better, and we educate patients and their families about that. In fact, not only is this notion false, but some drugs can have paradoxical effects when administered in high doses or for long periods of time, or even idiosyncratic reactions that are not necessarily dose related.

For example, psychostimulants like Adderall and Ritalin that are often used for children with ADHD can exacerbate anxiety and flatten affect or personality—that is, lead to the appearance of lethargy or lack of interest—even while improving focus and attention. Parents sometimes ask to have their children switched off these drugs because it removes their sense of joy.

Selective serotonin reuptake inhibitors (SSRIs), used for depression, anxiety, and obsessive-compulsive disorders, and antiepileptic drugs, used to achieve behavioral stabilization, can cause disinhibition, or unrestrained, "activated" behavior, much like someone with bipolar disorder experiencing mania. In fact, it is generally true that drugs used for behavioral stabilization and control can cause paradoxical worsening of behavior, sometimes dose related, sometimes idiosyncratic. Antidepressants, antianxiety drugs, certain antiepileptic drugs, and some other drug classes can cause thoughts of doing self-harm and even suicidal thinking, with concerns that some may actualize these thoughts. This gives physicians second thoughts about using these drugs, although they are the very medications designed for the neuropsychiatric issues afflicting many of the patients we see. Thus is the paradox within the paradox: the medications specifically designed for the disorders we treat can impose antagonistic effects and therefore limit our ability to prescribe them.

After we have monitored a patient for a sufficient period of time and found they are tolerating prescribed medications, if there are suboptimal benefits, we might elect to increase the dose, if necessary, to optimize improvements. Even then, we remain true to the "Start low; go slow" philosophy.

> **The medications specifically designed for the disorders we treat can impose antagonistic effects and therefore limit our ability to prescribe them.**

Increasing doses in irresponsible increments that produce serious side effects is more than just counterproductive from a treatment standpoint; it can demoralize patients and their family, potentially reducing their commitment and compliance with the regimen. From the perspective of everyone involved, a low and slow pharmacological philosophy is a wise investment of time and understanding that pays off in happier, healthier patients and their families, even if the treatment effects might take a little longer.

I will share a testimonial that highlights the benefits of the "Start low; go slow" methodology. Jack came to us at age twelve after nine years of treatment for autism and associated issues. He was on a series of medications, including the antidepressant Zoloft (sertraline) to treat depression and anxiety. Jack's symptoms were well controlled with the drug, but he had become obese and lethargic, common side effects of many antidepressants and antipsychotics (also known as neuroleptics). Our low and slow methodology works in reverse as well, and we began slowly weaning Jack off the Zoloft.

As we reduced his dosage, we carefully monitored his condition and quickly observed that there didn't appear to be any discernible worsening of his mental state. By the time we had titrated the drug to half his previous dose, we were able to observe a reduction in side effects. Jack was losing weight and becoming more engaged and engaging. We continued to notch down the dosage with careful monitoring without any impact on Jack's mental state. By the time we had cut his prescription to one-quarter its original dosage without any increase in symptoms, Jack had returned to normal weight and was exhibiting a mischievous streak that had been absent when he arrived.

It was as if Jack had spent much of his early life with his personality stored away in the pillbox just waiting for us to free it.

We continue to provide ABA and other therapies for his autism and kept him on the lowest dosage of Zoloft necessary to prevent a relapse of depression but found ourselves treating an entirely new boy. Jack is much more involved in his own therapy, and his educators in school report he is better accepted by his peers because of his more typical affect and weight. This is an illustration of the medicine controlling one problem while creating another, and the need for considering periodic "medication reversals" if there are adverse side effects, or to reassess the need and efficacy of medications being given over long periods of time. We were able to find a middle ground that eliminated the new problem without affecting the management of the original one.

Note that I have described the pharmacological element of treatment as *part* of a therapeutic regimen. Medications are generally an adjunct to our treatment plan, and can reinforce or facilitate the medical, behavior, art, music, psychological, and other therapies we administer. There are cases where medications are the most effective part of a treatment regimen, other cases where nonpharmacological interventions are dominant, and still other cases where the combination is the best approach.

Drugs are like the vice president of our treatment plan: an important part of the government but rarely the leader. On occasions, when the president is traveling overseas or hospitalized, the VP may handle presidential duties, just

> **Drugs are like the vice president of our treatment plan: an important part of the government but rarely the leader.**

as drugs may occasionally take the lead when appropriate. But in both cases, that is the exception rather than the rule.

OUR PATIENTS' DECLARATIONS OF INDEPENDENCE

It is common to view the few differences between the neurotypical majority and individuals on the autism spectrum, or those with other neurological disorders, rather than focus on the many attributes that all humans share. As adults, those with autism spectrum disorder need to carry out the activities of daily living, work, go to school, develop relationships, and build lives, just as anyone else does. Independence can pose challenges for individuals with autism spectrum disorder due to the nature of the disorder and deficits in executive function.

Many individuals with autism suffer poor long-term outcomes as adults in self-care, education, employment, health, living arrangements, and relationship building. The optimized outcome for high-functioning individuals on the spectrum is to achieve full independence; for others, it may include lower levels of independence, like living in a structured setting and holding a structured job that requires some independent work skills. For others still, whose symptoms are more severe, the long-term goals may be even more humble within the rubric of complete or near-complete dependence.

Nurturing independence is an iterative process built into treatment plans over a patient's entire childhood and even into adulthood. A variety of strategies can be employed to build independence, starting with giving children with autism choices. This can be as small as choosing which game to play, which snack to eat, or which activity to engage in. Children with autism are most likely to develop a sense of self-reliance when everyone in their life allows them to make decisions of increasing importance as they age. This includes parents, siblings, teachers, therapists, and doctors.

Educators, therapists, and parents are encouraged to help build this desire and ability one step at a time. For example, a child who likes apple juice might first be encouraged to indicate they want a drink using language—oral or sign, or by exchanging a picture of a drink. After they have mastered that, they might be encouraged to get their cup as the indicator. The next stop might be the caregiver and child pouring the apple juice into the cup together and, finally, the child going to the refrigerator and pouring it for themselves. The learning process will not be linear—juice will be spilled—but the sense of empowerment and self-reliance the child will feel as he masters each step will foster the desire to continue and achieve that one data point of independence.

Matt's story at the beginning of this chapter is a quintessential example of the life-changing nature of achieving independence. Matt is not autistic, but his vomiting disorder and all its accompanying dyspepsia and misery were poised to disrupt his life, interfering with his education, family, and social life and threatening the ability to become an independent adult. Relieving his condition has given him back his life, as his parents have noted to us.

The ability to live a quality life without relying on others is an optimized outcome—perhaps the ultimate one for those with neurological, neurodevelopmental, and neurobehavioral disorders—but it takes time to reveal itself in full. All children are dependent on their parents, teachers, and other adults, to one degree or another. Nonetheless, the development of independence in the context of childhood is visible and measurable.

When Maryanne talks about the two sons she brought to us, she focuses mostly on the process I have described in detail here—the comprehensive assessment beyond anything she had experienced anywhere else; the way doctors and therapists genuinely listened to her; the comprehensive services in one facility; the integrated medical care her children received from a pediatric neurologist, a behavioral pediatrician, and a neuropsychologist; and the integration of their work with the behaviorists, therapists, and the rest of the staff. We appreciate her satisfaction with our service, of course, but all of that would be moot if we had failed to put her children on a path toward independence.

The assessment of Maryanne's autistic teenage son, Ryan, determined that he was on the wrong medications, so new meds were prescribed, and "that turned his behavior around," she said.

Our behaviorists provided him with tools to manage situations and put him in art therapy with his neurotypical teen sister, with whom he had a rocky relationship. They worked together on a project that helped them learn to communicate with each other.

"I love it when I go home and see my daughter try to respond to him the same way he is responding to her. They're communicating, and they're getting over that bridge," she said.

Ryan's path to independence is clear now that he is using the tools he needs to take care of himself and develop relationships with those around him.

We have adult patients with autism originally brought to us as children by parents despairing that they could never live quality lives without a lifetime of supervision and guidance but who now live independently, are employed, and are married parents themselves. This is the pinnacle of optimized outcomes, of course, but the only path there is years of optimized short-term outcomes that help erect the foundation of a functional life rather than check boxes without any practical relevance to the life of the individual.

As I've mentioned, healthcare in the United States generally, and in particular for neurobehavioral and related disorders, is not cost-effective, can lack precision, is dependent on pharmaceuticals, often results in avoidable hospital and institutional care, and lacks strategies for disease prevention. Much is changing in healthcare, and much is being discussed about how to make healthcare work for the individual seeking care.

In the next chapter, we will discuss how that is possible—because it is already happening. The odds against us remain great, the vested interests remain entrenched and powerful, and the inertia is as difficult to overcome as ever. But there is a blueprint for a functioning and cost-effective healthcare delivery system for those with special needs such as autism, and we will discuss it.

CHAPTER 5

First, There Is Hope ...

Imagine walking into our offices at NeurAbilities Healthcare seeking answers to the concerning behavior of your two-year-old son. You remember the joy that his birth and infancy brought you, but the subsequent few months have tempered that emotion. You know something is wrong, but you can't put your finger on it. You come to us seeking answers.

After a thorough evaluation and neurodiagnostic testing, we have distressing news: your child has moderate to severe autism, a chronic neurological disorder that can severely limit his ability to function. This news shatters your idealized dreams of family life; it will not be "typical" from here on in. The "typical" developmental milestones that other families measure their children against may have little meaning in your household; you will need to find new ways to accommodate and celebrate your child.

Initially, you and your spouse may be overwhelmed by a new diagnosis. We educate you about the diagnosis, its meaning and implications, and that there are various treatment approaches available once we have a clinical and biological profile of your child. It will take continued effort and hard work to propel your child to his full potential, whatever that might ultimately encompass.

And, perhaps, the most difficult aspect of this diagnosis is this: we cannot forecast how your child will perform long term.

Maybe he will be one of the minority of children who "recover" from an early autism diagnosis and become relatively indistinguishable from neurotypical peers. Or, in the case of severe autism, he will need full supports for activities of daily living and, depending on co-occurring conditions, will have a shortened life expectancy. In cases of mild autism, your child will have to learn some coping strategies to avoid social awkwardness but can enjoy life and become an independent and successful adult. Many determinants will contribute to where on that spectrum your child may fall.

Though our clinicians diagnose patients with autism daily, it does not get any easier. We guide our patients and their families through their grief and acceptance journey. We help them with building resilience and instill confidence in planning for any challenge, while appreciating the joys a special needs child can bring to a family. We offer realistic expectations that ensure a practical path forward. And with compassion and empathy we share our straightforward assessments and offer hope for the future.

As our CEO, Kathleen Bailey Stengel, keeps reminding us: we give families five minutes to cry. Their grief is real and understandable, but they will have their whole lives to endure that emotional process. After five minutes, it is time to roll up our sleeves and get to work. The science demonstrates quite clearly that the earlier treatment begins, the better the results.

Most families appreciate our approach. Many have done their own research and are well prepared for the diagnosis they receive. Autism is expressed externally, so they already know there is a problem and very often have internalized the possibility of this finding. They may not be surprised at all and are ready for whatever is next and eager to move forward. On the other hand, that may all be true, yet the definitiveness of the diagnosis is nonetheless shocking. In any case, once they get over the initial shock, families generally begin committing themselves to supporting their child and, if not quite ready to begin, are amenable to our determination to put their child on the right path.

One family that was not quite on board this way sticks in my memory. The family came to us after an unsatisfactory visit to a clinic to determine why their two-year-old girl was not developing like other children. We diagnosed the child with autism and recommended ABA therapy, an empirically recognized autism treatment. Every child is unique and will have their own path, but ABA therapy is almost always a lynchpin of early treatment.

When we broke the news, the entire family erupted in stage one of grief—denial. The grandmother broke down, refusing to believe the news. The father blamed the mother. Anger and recrimination flew about the room as the family struggled to cope with this traumatic news. Our therapist exited the room to allow the family to process that information in whatever way worked for them. After five minutes (we say five, but that is metaphorical), they simply needed to take a breath to internalize the consequences of the information they had received.

Our therapist returned and put a halt to the disagreements. She reminded the family that autism is a condition, not a fatal disease, and refuted in no uncertain terms the notion that their daughter's condition was anyone's "fault." She told them it was time to take positive steps forward for the sake of their child and reminded them, as we always do, of the uncertainty of the future and of our commitment to the best possible outcome.

The family settled down and agreed that their catharsis was complete, and they were ready to begin acting in the best interests of their child.

It is at this point in the case that instigated this discussion, when you have brought your two-year-old child in and received an autism diagnosis, that we offer you the one thing you need most: hope.

Not unrealistic hope, because we truly don't know what the future will bring, but the persistent hope that is nestled in the knowledge that there is a team of experts supporting you; working relentlessly; never giving up; committed to the best interests of your child and your family; melding science with a heart for our patients; and treating your child as a whole, unique individual and not as a diagnosis.

Hope is ubiquitous and omnipresent because the future can change. Your child's brain can surprise us, a developmental growth spurt can occur at age three or four, and new discoveries can alter the landscape. After all, we remain in the infancy of autism neurobiological research. Our understanding of the condition remains primitive, and yet it is a thousand times more advanced than it was twenty years ago and infinitely better than it was in the 1960s when some eminences in the field were declaring that autism was the fault of frigid and heartless mothers.

> **Hope is ubiquitous and omnipresent because the future can change.**

We have seen several inflection points of progress in the treatment of autism, including proof of the efficacy of behavioral therapy; recognition that autism is a spectrum and that each child has their own individual set of strengths, deficits, and behaviors; and most recently, the explosion of understanding around the genetic mechanisms and other biological causes and contributions affecting autism. Genetics is likely to represent the area of greatest advancement in our comprehension and treatment of autism for the near future, especially if not from an acquired environmental, immunological, or other organic insult to brain development or organization.

If your child is engaged in therapy, particularly with providers like us eager to adopt cutting-edge techniques, any advances in the science hold the possibility of benefiting them. So we offer all our patients— parents as well as children—a dollop of hope alongside the hard work of evaluation, diagnosis, treatment, outcome measurement, and daily reinforcement. It can only be accomplished through the daily grind of good parenting that courageously navigates the challenging needs and requirements of autism but with a view toward the horizon and the hope that a breakthrough may accelerate the value of everything we do today.

So Kathleen will tell you that your grief is real, and you have five minutes to cry about this news. But then, we need to get to work. Because there is hope.

THEN, THE JOURNEY

"A goal without a plan is just a wish," allegedly said the twentieth-century author Antoine de Saint-Exupéry.

Hope is necessary but insufficient on its own for our families. Next, we provide them with a plan. We sketch out for the family in broad terms what their journey will look like and have even produced modeling videos to train them. The journey begins with a meeting for further assessments because simply determining that a child has autism has little value.

Parents have all the *W* questions: who, what, when, where, why (and how, which inconveniently does not start with a *W*). Imagine your orthopedist diagnosing your shoulder issues as a torn rotator cuff, shaking your hand, and wishing you a good day. That would hardly be useful or actionable. Our assessments begin to examine the contours and intensity of a child's autism, delve into comorbidities, explore for biological causes, and examine the shape, intensity, and frequency of dysfunctional behaviors.

We employ objective tools and clinical information to provide more detail to the diagnosis and clinical profile. That might include the Autism Diagnostic Observation Schedule (ADOS, now in a second edition: ADOS-2), an empirical, observational test that is normed and scored to provide objective information for categorization of autism, augmented by a structured interview with the Autism Diagnostic Inventory-Revised (ADI-R). This information allows for classification and categorization of a severe, moderate, or mild form of autism and for defining associated developmental, clinical, and environmental problems.

At this point, we are providing materials to the parents to coordinate with childcare providers and schools because children do not spend most of their time in our office; if they attend childcare or school, they will spend much more time there. Our staff's main function in preparing the family for their coming journey is to serve as Sherpas, guiding the family up the mountain over treacherous terrain while assuring them about the appropriate paths to get to the top. But we haven't gone up their child's particular mountain and don't know what their peak looks like. We are experienced guides, but we have never ventured up the same mountain twice.

> **But we haven't gone up their child's particular mountain and don't know what their peak looks like. We are experienced guides, but we have never ventured up the same mountain twice.**

In the first year, our approach tends to be more fluid and subject to course correction for the obvious reason that each child's case is unique. We spend that first year collecting and analyzing information across a wide array of functions and get more precise as we move forward. Because autism isn't the result of one thing but rather a set of maladaptive behaviors, developmental impairments, and neurological and medical conditions, we address the symptoms and signs instead of generically treating "autism."

We intervene immediately when we know there is a need—say, in language development—without necessarily having an immediate precision diagnosis. The longer we work with a child, the more precise the diagnoses and the more finely tuned, more tailored, the treatment plan. One thing we know is that any child's treatment plan will be different from every other's because, as we chant like a mantra, if you've seen one child with autism, you've seen one child with autism.

AN OVERNIGHT SUCCESS (TWENTY YEARS IN THE MAKING)

At NeurAbilities, we truly believe we have a frame-breaking concept, a better way to deliver services to a vulnerable population and something worth writing about and emulating throughout the health-care system. We have something that transcends an idea, and we have worked on proof of this concept for the better part of two decades. We have fashioned a practice that succeeds in creating an innovative and unique healthcare delivery and clinical model that is providing quality care, positive experiences, and successful outcomes. Although we must presently function within the fee-for-service environment, our model is equipped and ready to thrive in evolving systems of care and alternative payment models. Fee-for-service has proven to create unnecessary barriers, burdens, and flawed economic incentives that can be overcome with alternative reimbursement systems that reward value rather than disvalue, quality over quantity, and meaningful outcomes. Our solution to this conundrum is an inter-disciplinary, synergistic, holistic, independent, and diagnosis-agnostic clinical model that focuses on understanding the biological causes and contributions to the disorders and diseases circumscribing the lives of our patients while delivering personalized precision treatment strategies and regimens. We believe our model is worth real investigation, experimentation, and evaluation because it shows promise for being better for our patients, their families, and all the other stakeholders in their lives. I began with this seed of an idea fueled by my medical experience in the crucible of the AIDS epidemic and honed by (now) over thirty years of medical practice in academic, hospital, nonprofit organizations, and independent/private practice settings. We have tested, learned, shaped, and improved the implementation of this idea and continue to. Our journey as an independent organization began in 2005, and soon after the Great Recession of 2008 cast its shadow. With persistence and perseverance, and an attitude that failure was not an option, we continued to grow exponentially despite the challenges because of the acute need for our services and our viable solution and desirable alternative.

How did we grow organically without outside investment? By focusing on our mission and vision predicated on delivering quality clinical services matching our core value of compassionate care. By emphasizing quality over quantity with a willingness to take financial risks to serve our patients. By bridging gaps in the healthcare system and meeting the needs of every patient. It was a big leap, particularly in the shadow of five of the largest pediatric institutions and hospital systems in the country in the southern New Jersey/Philadelphia area.

We are not unique in offering comprehensive services, but our difference is how we deliver these services and our focus on improving our Specialty Care Medical Home model. We knew the risks were high and odds for success daunting. In the region of the nation with the highest incidence of autism, we knew the challenge would not be about finding demand for our services but about meeting those needs while remaining fiscally viable. There was a void in meeting those needs as comprehensively, effectively, efficiently, independently, collaboratively, holistically, or precisely as we do. We recognized the need for our services, but could we navigate the regulatory, compliance, and business issues? In other words, we were well positioned in the areas we could control and totally at risk in the areas we could not control.

No wonder few others were taking the leap we took.

There were points where we were on the brink and knew we might not survive, especially during the Great Recession of 2008, shortly after the beginning of our journey. But the financial and other challenges strengthened our resolve as failure was not a viable option for the patients and families we serve. And the lessons learned during that era taught us how to create more sustainable business systems. We emerged stronger and continued to grow and scale our operations over tenfold during the first thirteen years of existence.

The year 2018 was a very important inflection point in our history. We recognized that getting to the next level would require additional financial resources and management expertise. Thus, we made the decision to partner with the Council Capital investment group.

If you are first hearing about us, it is tempting to consider our enterprise as new, our success nascent. We are like an actor hailed for their "breakthrough" performance in a popular movie after twenty years of honing their craft in local theater and off-Broadway—an overnight sensation who has been practicing and preparing for two decades.

We see ourselves as positive disruptors in an industry much more resistant to change, beholden to government and third-party payers, glacial in its acceptance of innovations, opaque and sclerotic. We have been beset by obstacles—not just in perfecting the implementation of our concept but in battling with the underlying conditions inherent in a healthcare system that is resistant to change, innovation, and disruption and slow to recognize our model's utility and adoption.

As an independent organization of limited size, we needed better financial and administrative resources to deal with the modern-day realities of healthcare, such as extensive and expensive information technologies, regulatory and compliance issues, payer contracting and preauthorizations, billings and collections, human resources, payroll, marketing, legal consultation, infrastructure needs, and more.

And with the investment of Council Capital, we have been able to add many more clinicians, technicians, and administrative and support staff, and added many more facilities throughout our expanding multistate presence: from the humble beginnings of one small office and a handful of employees to now eighteen facilities and four hundred plus employees. We have shown that our model is replicable and sustainable. We have exceeded a proof of concept and created a thriving reality. The healthcare system is beginning to take notice as we accelerate our growth in making our care delivery model accessible to different regions of ever-larger segments of special needs populations and countless more with other neurological disabilities, delivering clinical benefits with a proven approach to diagnosing and treating their conditions and disorders.

HOW TO BE A CUTTING-EDGE DINOSAUR

We pride ourselves on operating at the forefront of healthcare, innovating in ways we believe, or at least hope, will be commonplace in the foreseeable future. We also pride ourselves on our ability to see what is coming, and what is needed, by taking the pulse of the community at large; we are in the field in the thick of the battle—on the front lines, not observing from an ivory tower. That puts us ahead of the curve, yet in a very real and inopportune way, we are also dinosaurs, relics of a glorious past. The big shift in the last few decades in managed care and consolidation among hospitals and healthcare systems has been the corporatization of healthcare. These large systems, driven by cost control and revenue enhancement, are squeezing out smaller providers, gobbling up independent physician practices like Pac-Man characters. That has left fewer and fewer independent practices committed to the best interests of patients and not to the agendas and demands of corporate and institutional entities. Although the goal of consolidation of healthcare into large, hospital-based systems was an attempt to reduce costs through economies of scale, there have been negative consequences as well, particularly for those who need to provide the care.

A 2018 survey by the Physicians Foundation found more than half of physicians suffering "very negative" morale, nearly two-thirds pessimistic about the future, three-quarters experiencing burnout "often or always," and fewer than one in five confident that the reimbursement structure is beneficial to patients.[36] Just 5 percent of physicians said the best approach to healthcare in the United States is to maintain the current system. As previously discussed, in my own field of child neurology, I was part of a task force that reported on the attitude of the clinical workforce in 2015, finding widespread dissatisfactions because of mounting regulatory and administrative stresses interfering with clinical practice, raising fears that these can be barriers for recruitment of new trainees into a specialty already in high demand with a critical shortage of child neurologists.[37]

I also participated on a task force convened in 2017 by the Child Neurology Society, again finding high levels of physician burnout

---

36   Merritt Hawkins, "2018 Survey of America's Physicians: Practice Patterns and Perspectives," The Physicians Foundation, accessed March 9, 2023, https://physiciansfoundation.org/wp-content/uploads/2018/09/physicians-survey-results-final-2018.pdf.

37   Kang et. al, "The Child Neurology Clinical Workforce."

approaching 90 percent for those working in academic and hospital-based institutions, characterized by emotional exhaustion, depersonalization (feelings of cynicism and detachment), and a sense of ineffectiveness at work (low sense of personal accomplishment). However, child neurologists working within independent organizations and practices had higher rates of satisfaction compared to those within institutions. The task force concluded that there is a need for innovation, alternative payment models, value-based medicine approaches, and practice efficiencies.[38, 39]

These issues should be concerning to everyone, not just physicians. A strong and available healthcare force is necessary for society, but if healthcare provider burnout is not addressed and dissatisfaction reversed, what has been a premier healthcare system will be diminished, and patients will suffer.

As I noted in chapter 3, the roots of our fragmented healthcare system can be traced to World War II, when unions negotiated for benefits like free health insurance during a time of wage and price controls. By the 1980s, insurers were scrambling to manage costs and created a managed care system, in which care is delivered by a network of providers complying with prearranged rules and reimbursed in a codified manner. Payment mechanisms that required approvals for nearly every healthcare service were established, igniting the ire of both providers and patients who rebelled against these constraints. Costs continued to rise, and clinical outcomes declined as care was restricted for cost considerations.

The managed care model has morphed alongside the emergence of the healthcare megasystems in the past two decades. There is greater

---

38 Kerry Levin et al., "Burnout, Career Satisfaction, and Well-Being among US Neurology Residents and Fellows in 2016," *Neurology* 89, no. 5 (2017): 492–501, doi:10.1212/ WNL.0000000000004135.

39 Zupanc, "Child Neurology in the 21st Century," 2020.

flexibility for patients and providers, but reimbursement for health-care services remains siloed, and, therefore, so do the services them-selves. We are not alone advocating for a more rational and effective reimbursement system that bundles services into a coherent set of treatments. We have presented to some payers about our alternative payment model proposals that focus on outcomes and value.

Right from the start in 2005, we determined to go in a different direction. As healthcare was rapidly consolidating, we chose indepen-dence. Our services do not depend on a hospital system, government, or other bureaucratic entity. Nevertheless, we often collaborate with hospitals, clinics, schools, and government to secure the comprehen-sive services our patients need across their entire lives and not just when they visit our offices. Our value-based care is holistic from the moment patients and their families walk in the door until they no longer need our services.

As pioneers, we attempt to bring the healthcare system closer to adopting integrated innovation in the service of patients and their families. We have worked within the present fee-for-service reimburse-ment system to bring many of the services our patients need under one roof. You can call it value-based care or risk-based reimbursement or bundled services, but at the end of the day, it's just the care our patients need—provided by an interdisciplinary team of experts in a single medical home that manages the array of services required by the patient wherever they go, free from the strangling bureaucracies, agnostic about diagnoses, and focused only on achieving the best outcomes. For autistic children who comprise a significant percentage of our patients, that means successful inclusion into social and educational systems and as close to living independently as they can get as they become adults.

The components of patient-centered medical homes for autism have recently been published by Dr. Michael Cameron of the University of Southern California.[40] His group has outlined that an effective medical home will provide comprehensive care, including ASD screening and diagnostic services; provide specialty medical care, ABA, and other therapies; have the ability to provide services in the home; collaborate with patients, families, and schools; be accessible; provide adolescent-to-adult transition programs; coordinate interdisciplinary care; and strive for high-quality care. Our Specialty Care Medical Home model of healthcare delivery for special needs populations meets these criteria, and thus, we are well positioned for the future of value-based care and alternative payment models.

"The service delivery system is poised for a paradigm shift—specifically, a shift from a fragmented approach to treatment-centered around maximizing billing hours, to an approach guided by a patient-centered medical home model that focuses on the client and their family, optimizes access to treatment, prioritizes interdisciplinary collaboration and coordination of care, monitors efficiency, ensures the safeguarding of clients, uses established outcome measures to evaluate the effectiveness of treatment, delivers culturally competent care, and ensures an integrated approach to treatment," he writes.

You can't attend a seminar or convention in our industry without hearing multiple references to innovations that produce superior outcomes. These presentations come complete with empirical data and PowerPoints graphically depicting one theory of care delivery or another. We have something else: a model of care that works and produces optimized outcomes for our patients in a more cost-effective way.

Our proof isn't in a PowerPoint deck or a well-researched theory: it is on the front lines of the patients we have assessed with cutting-

---

40   Yiftah Frechter et al., "Toward a Value-Based Care Model for Children with Autism Spectrum Disorder," *Open Access Journal of Behavioural & Science Psychology* 5, no. 1 (2022): 180065, https://www.academicstrive.com/OAJBSP/OAJBSP180065.pdf.

edge tools and treated inter- and transdisciplinarily, whose care we have managed, and whose symptoms and behaviors have improved after years of stagnation prior to finding us. Our methods require up-front comprehensive evaluations and a modicum of patience. Our approaches reduce fragmentation of care, lessen utilization of expensive hospital-based resources, and eschew pharmaceuticals when nonpharmaceutical therapies can suffice. That is the message we bring to payers: our methods appear extravagant, but they actually reduce the overall cost of care.

And the cost of care for autism is staggering. There are estimates that the lifetime societal cost for an individual with ASD is $3.6 million, and with the increasing number of new cases, a total of $4 trillion over the next decade—and possibly up to $15 trillion if the rate of increase in prevalence continues. For perspective, the total US government federal revenue for 2021 was approximately $4 trillion.[41]

How could an insurer, whether private or government insurance, possibly conceptualize the long-term benefit of our integrated services when they have divided healthcare into quanta of services, distinct bits of care valued and delivered separately from every other bit of care? They are counting the trees, and we are looking at the forest. They are focused on the bits of quantifiable service delivered, and we are focused on the patient and their experiences. They tend to focus on short-term benefits, whereas we are targeting both short-term improvement as well as long-term outcomes. We have had to show them that our way is better, overcome the inertia of the system, and create change. It has been a struggle.

We have reengineered the diagnosis process and avoided pigeon-holing people into a single diagnosis—for example, autism—and

---

41   Janet Cakir et al., "The Lifetime Social Cost of Autism: 1990–2029," *Research in Autism Spectrum Disorders* 72 (April 2020): 101502, https://doi.org/10.1016/j.rasd.2019.101502.

instead think about them from a biological, behavioral, neuropsy-chological, and clinical standpoint. We view our patients not just as a biological species—though that is an aspect of all of us—but also as humans, examining the full array of humanistic qualities to get those optimized outcomes. What does that mean to our entrenched health-care system that is dependent on diagnostic and procedure codes and productivity measured by volume rather than outcomes?

Kathleen Bailey Stengel regales healthcare colleagues with her opening impression of our company. The day she assumed her position, she heard me on the phone with an insurer, battling to get reimburse-ment for our services. The insurer was denying a metaphorical nickel of our claim. They were fighting with us over a nickel. They knew that no one in his right mind would bother to engage in a protracted skirmish over five cents, so they could just slice that five cents off every claim and grind every provider into submission. Eventually, they could produce a system where providers were self-censoring over the nickel, and just to be sure, the next dime, until they challenged a quarter, then a half dollar, and eventually one hundred dollars on every claim.

This war of attrition exhausts providers and convinces them to absorb the loss or reduce the service they provide rather than engage in endless combat—at great cost in time and productivity—with each of the many insurance companies and payers. That is what a practice in its right mind would do, but no one in their right mind would have done what we did in the first place: take on the quixotic venture of starting a healthcare organization insisting on productive innovation.

Driving innovation in healthcare while disrupting an entrenched system is emotionally and cognitively draining. This is not like Uber or Amazon, which can create disruptive technology that attracts paying customers and eviscerates the taxicab and retail industries respectively. In healthcare, we are paid, not directly by the consumers who flock to us, but by this Byzantine web of commercial and government insurers, and other payers, who have been empowered to decide what care may be delivered and how much to pay for it. Our innovative approach to neurohealth requires adequate coverage for its costs. Thus, Kathleen walked into our offices on her first day of work and heard the founder of the company and its chief medical officer refusing to concede that even one-twentieth of a dollar of our services was unnecessary, because it wasn't, because our methods are demonstrably better for patients, providers, and the system, and because we refuse to set a precedent that will rob our practice of its edge. She must have had second thoughts at that moment about the wisdom of her decision to embark on this new adventure, but fortunately for all of us, she stuck with us.

We have had many conversations with insurers, presenting our model and our outcomes, and they have found it consonant with their movement toward value-based healthcare delivery. Insurers are not opposed to change that can reduce their costs in the long run. But they don't know how to fit our square peg into the round holes that characterize the entirety of the healthcare system. Here is a case in point: we have asked the insurance companies for metrics against which we could benchmark our services. That is, *What does long-term outcome X cost to deliver in total, and how often is it achieved?* The insurers couldn't tell us. They are not even measuring long-term outcomes because no one is thinking about them and because people switch insurance companies all the time, so there is little point in concerning themselves about whether an autistic child can live on their own and get a job. They are interested instead in short-term outcomes, like whether the child can learn to follow a direction or ask for a drink of water, because that is easy to measure.

Consider this scenario and the insurance response to it: a child is diagnosed with autism and prescribed twenty-five hours a week of ABA therapy. Intensive ABA therapy is likely to be part of the prescription for any autistic child because it has a history of empirical success and is considered the gold standard for behavioral treatment. Based on a detailed skills assessment and a functional behavior assessment, children are prescribed direct services to increase skills and reduce or remediate problematic behaviors. In general, these hours are derived from a clinical impression and average set of needs for a child with similar deficits.

As you can already discern yourself, the child in question may or may not be "average," even within the community of those with autism. He or she might have concurrent physical problems, comorbidities, a shorter or longer attention span, more or less stamina than average, etc. This is not a very precise prescription, but it is reasonable and likely to be authorized by payers. We assert that a much more extensive assessment is necessary to determine the unique circumstances of each child, to reveal etiology that is not apparent and may not be affected by behavioral therapy, to focus on the specific behaviors of the child and determine, with much more precision, how much and what kind of therapy he or she needs. Our personalized prescription does not readily conform to preauthorization requirements, as payer policies do not necessarily comport with patient needs. But payers are beginning to understand that our approach provides value to both patient and payer and thus can create a "win-win" situation.

How do we know our methods are succeeding? The answer is existential: we have not only remained in business, but we have also thrived. We have negotiated rates with insurers that have allowed us to continue to deliver care according to our vision and ethos because they understand that the patients we serve are part of a very difficult population to manage, yet their own data demonstrates that we do it well. Insurers want to apply the same methods to pay for autism services that they use to pay for knee replacement, even while the differences are stark. Knee replacement surgery is less complex to create a bundled payment, as the event is episodic, limited, with defined outcomes, and very anatomically focused.

But autism services—at least the way we provide them—are too complex for linear thinking. A neurologist, pediatric psychologist, medical geneticist, and a host of others contribute their expertise—not in discrete bursts but in an integrated effort to assess, diagnose, treat, and measure our patients over their entire childhood and sometimes beyond. The nuances of our work often escape the grasp of those beholden to the current system, but we continue to chip away at the entrenched bureaucracy. As we have presented and has been published, alternative payment and value-based models are urgently needed for autism and related conditions. We have confidence that eventually, our ideas will be considered conventional wisdom.

> **The nuances of our work often escape the grasp of those beholden to the current system, but we continue to chip away at the entrenched bureaucracy.**

I want to be clear that we do not believe that we have all the answers or have solved all the problems in neurohealth care. Our processes, diagnoses, assessments, evaluations, treatments, and execution continue to improve. Though we aim to help every patient, we may not succeed with all. Still, we evaluate any shortcomings and reexamine our methodologies often. We discuss and debate internally how to improve every aspect of our work on a weekly basis, and we know we will never reach a conclusion because even if we were ever to perfect it all, which is not possible, something would change the next day and require new solutions. We are continuously seeking to improve the quality of our practice all the time. But perfection is not the standard—improvement is, and we can see that what we have created and operationalized for nearly two decades is an improvement over the status quo.

WHY WRITE A BOOK?

I did not set out to write a book depicting my view of a reimagined healthcare system in hopes that others would adopt it. Instead, Pnina and I gathered a like-minded team and built this reimagined healthcare delivery system first and made it work. We haven't just theorized that the silos could be knocked down; we knocked them down. We haven't merely postulated that we could operate independently under the withering gaze of many pediatric hospital Goliaths; we have operated independently. We haven't simply believed that an integrated, holistic, diagnosis-agnostic approach to neurological disorders could produce better outcomes; we have executed that idea and produced superior outcomes for nearly two decades.

Only then did I embark on writing a book—not about a theory for others to adopt but about a theory we adopted and proved can work. It has been frustrating to demonstrate a formula that delivers superior outcomes to patients in need of neurological and other services and discover that not only has it not achieved widespread adoption, but it remains the anomaly. We hear many questions about many aspects of healthcare, especially for our population of patients, but we don't hear many concrete solutions. We have provided a concrete solution, and the response from the marketplace has been consistent growth. The response from inside the healthcare system has been lacking. Change is hard, and entrenched interests are slow to acknowledge that the established methods may require change and innovation. The proliferation of our model cannot happen without a reimbursement system that supports it; otherwise, the next wave of practitioners will find themselves tilting at the same windmills, fighting the same battles, breaking the same ground that we already have.

We hope others adopt our methods—not because the idea is intriguing but because autistic children and others with neurological disorders would benefit from it. We know that because we have already produced and tested the blueprint. We hope to expand our practice beyond its current scope, but we cannot do this alone. Witnessing a surge in similar practices throughout the country would fulfill us professionally because it would amount to tacit admission that we developed an innovation and provide hope to thousands more individuals desperately in need of hope.

After thirteen years of organic growth, in order to catapult our business to the exponential growth that the market suggests is awaiting us, we began considering further growth strategies in 2018. We had taken our business about as far as a dedicated contingent of doctors, psychologists, therapists, and administrative and support staff could, but how could we bring on business partners of one type or another when health insurers and government healthcare policy experts struggle to comprehend our model? How do we maintain our independence from bureaucracy if we engaged a corporate entity?

These and more questions were answered when Council Capital approached us, unbidden, to combine forces. They would provide their professional business and management expertise and inject an infusion of capital, and we would present our frame-breaking ethos to interested parties. Frankly, we were somewhat tentative about the idea of joining forces with a private equity investment group.

We obsess about patients; private equity groups obsess about the bottom line. We jealously guard our independence; professional managers want control. We value customized care; businesspeople seek to streamline operations by standardizing and then replicating them.

We are complicated, with multiple disciplines at work, and even within the medical discipline, we provide niche specialty services—private equity searches for blueprints that can be exported to the next market.

But in our courtship with Council Capital, we found out something else about enlightened private equity firms like this one: they love innovation; they seek it out; they want to fund it. Thus, our goals and vision were aligned. In short, there is a market inefficiency for the joy and hope that our approach provides, and this enlightened private equity group latched onto it. They recognize the value that often eludes insurance companies and government entities because private equity firms are not stuck in a system that dampens innovation and enforces irrational and counterproductive practices for no reason other than that is the way they are done.

Eventually, Council Capital allayed our hesitations and presented us with ideas that could professionalize our management structure and operations without endangering our professional judgments, patient care, or customer service; indeed, their contributions would improve our service by making it more efficient and streamlining the customer experience. Not long after we signed the papers, they discovered the resilience of our operation. Like all in healthcare, in 2020 COVID-19 upended everything we do. Many hospitals turned most of their operations over to COVID-19 care while struggling to envision how they could treat other patients. Being a small, independent operation focused on a special needs population, we were able to shift the delivery of our services quickly to conform to COVID-19 pandemic realities. We embraced telehealth and maintained our patient focus, taking our services to our customers while maintaining our high standards of care.

Through this book, through our increased outreach, through a new commitment to growing and scaling what we have created, a new opportunity is arising for children and adults with autism spectrum and other neurological disorders, and for their parents, families, and other supporters. That opportunity requires a simple free-market concept to reconsider your status as "patients" and instead consider yourselves customers. As customers, you are used to demanding the best service at a reasonable price. Parents of children with autism should be demanding that their providers examine every aspect of their child and not merely hew to the standard treatment based on a broad diagnosis. They should be demanding integrated services from a community of disciplines; independence from large, bureaucratic institutions; coordination between the healthcare practitioners and schools; and case management from the specialist's office. In a free-market system, consumers get what they want. When autism customers—patients and their families—begin expecting the innovations that we have proven deliver superior outcomes for them, the system will finally begin to change.

That is the new challenge we have set for ourselves, not merely to continue delivering superior care via a Specialty Care Medical Home model of healthcare delivery but to change the entire system so that our model is the norm. Millions of families in this country struggling with autism and other neurological disorders should accept nothing less in order to expedite the change in healthcare services they deserve. That is our quest. It is a quest to provide hope for every child, adolescent, and adult on the spectrum or with other neurological disorders and neurodevelopmental disabilities—hope that whatever their ultimate potential, we will provide them a path to achieve it.

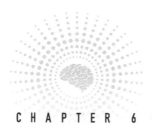

CHAPTER 6

A Clinical Model for Autism

et's recall the case of Chris, diagnosed early on in his life as autistic, with a host of comorbidities such as low muscle tone, constant fever, gastrointestinal issues, sleep disruption, and more. "He kind of got tagged as autistic," said his mother. "But there were always other things going on that I could never quite get answers to—until I came to NeurAbilities."

Chris had been stocked in the autism section of the healthcare supermarket, where he was labeled and put on the same shelf as all the other individuals similarly labeled. On that shelf, everyone is packaged and sold the same way—the same directions and warning information on each. As often happens with people who have neurodevelopmental or neuropsychiatric disorders, they are categorized in a broad diagnostic category with others who exhibit a certain set of behaviors and endure an array of related maladies; in Chris's case, he was stamped autistic and offered a standard set of nonindividualized treatments.

In other areas of medicine, knowledge and understanding of the biology of diseases has allowed for specific, individualized, "personalized," and "precision" interventions based on targeting the biological cause rather than only the clinical manifestations. For example, years ago, cancer patients were treated rather similarly with broad and rather toxic treatments such as chemotherapy and radiation that were marginally effective for the "average" patient. As a better understanding of the nature of cancers based on general clinical characteristics such as (organ) location and general histology (microscopic visualization of the cancer cell features) advanced, treatments became more specific and further progressed as histopathological techniques and other ways to identify and define biological features of cancer improved.

With the dawn of the genomic era, the ability to categorize cancer based on genetic variations and mutations precipitated major advances in the ability to provide individualized and personalized therapeutic regimens, which are now commonplace in the field of oncology. However, only recently are we recognizing that individuals with neurodevelopmental disabilities can be similarly characterized and categorized by their underlying biological phenotype and also be provided treatment regimens targeting underlying biological mechanisms of disease.

As you may recall, we looked beyond the diagnosis of autism spectrum disorder in Chris's case. Instead, we evaluated his behaviors and developed a unique narrative for him that required personalized treatment attuned to the exact nature of his condition. Because of the matrix of behaviors Chris was exhibiting, we performed several diagnostic tests, including HD-EEG, which discovered unusual brain wave activity that likely prompted some of his adverse behaviors. Additionally, genetic testing found a rare genetic disorder, and taken together—the neurological function and genetic disorder—we had drilled down diagnostically to an etiology that described him much more biologically and accurately than a heterogeneous and nonspecific "spectrum" disorder, informing us about treatment options that had not been previously considered. Our testing determined that Chris wasn't merely autistic, a cookie-cutter description that suggested he was like every other child with autism, but rather biologically unique.

We addressed each of Chris's issues separately and together, prescribing medication for some of the more easily controlled conditions and providing an integrated care plan that included a range of therapies for problematic and medication-unresponsive behaviors, and Chris's condition quickly and significantly improved. "Thank goodness he wasn't pigeonholed as only autistic [at NeurAbilities] because it turns out that's a small piece of him but that's not all of him," Evan told us.

To be clear, there is no silver bullet for Chris. Now, as a young adult, he continues to exhibit some of the behaviors and continues to struggle with some of the associated conditions that brought him to us. But we have never given up hope of continued improvement, and our staff has traveled along the path with the family every step of the way. "I can't describe in words how valuable that has been to us," Evan said.

Chris's journey is emblematic of the way autism spectrum disorders and related neurobehavioral and neurodevelopmental conditions can and should be assessed and treated. The study of the evolution in the diagnosis and treatment of autism is a lesson in the dangers of medical beliefs or doctrines that are not grounded in medical science. The early descriptions of autism suggested that autism was the result of childhood psychoses or defective parenting, most notably by mothers. This flawed conceptualization of autism spectrum disorders gave way to advances in medical science, which have established autism as a neurobiological disorder of early brain development.

There are many genetic, metabolic, hormonal, immunological, anatomical, toxicological, and physiological causes of autism spectrum disorders, as well as an array of gastrointestinal and other systemic issues that often accompany autism. Thus, individuals with ASD are a biologically heterogeneous population with extensive neurodiversity. Early identification and understanding of autism spectrum disorders are crucial because interventions at younger ages are associated with vastly improved outcomes.

The advent of understanding the biological subtypes of ASD, along with targeted medical therapies and coupled with a multifaceted therapeutic approach that encompasses behavioral, educational, social, speech, occupational, and other forms of therapies, has created a new and exciting era for individuals with ASD and related disorders and their families: personalized and precision medical care based upon clinical profiles and underlying biological subtypes.

Despite advances in diagnostic and therapeutic approaches, much of the care for individuals with autism, particularly children, is disjointed and siloed, and it is fodder to the whims of the health-care marketplace and its bizarre economics. Yet there are individuals and organizations beginning to steer this ship in a different direction in accordance with improved understanding of the disorders, their etiologies, and comorbidities, providing therapeutic care empirically demonstrated to guide neurodiverse individuals to a future as independent and productive as possible.

This new approach requires new ways of approaching ASD service delivery. It eschews suppression of symptoms in favor of understanding and treating the disorder. While a pill that temporarily addresses symptoms may deliver instant gratification and a measurable outcome at low cost, treatment that yields permanent behavior or developmental change is more durable and cost-effective, even if it involves more time, effort, and up-front costs.

This new approach is less iterative and more integrative; indeed, it is *wholly* integrative. It requires clinicians in many fields working collaboratively and sharing expertise from their unique perspectives.

It marries the expertise of physicians and nurses with the expertise of therapists to create a whole-child treatment plan. It transcends the clinical setting and accounts for a patient's life at home, at school, and beyond, because patients don't live in clinical settings or spend much of their day there. The new paradigm of service delivery to neurodiverse children establishes open lines of communication with educators and others in the child's school who will spend far more time with the child than will their physician or therapists.

The evolution in understanding autism over the past six decades has led to the recognition that autism is not a single disorder but a spectrum of disorders with associated medical, neurological, neurodevelopmental, and neuropsychiatric health issues that are, taken together, unique to each individual. Consequently, there is new recognition that treatment must be customized to each individual patient. This has led to a focus on precision medicine (i.e., based on the specifics of each patient and not on the "average" patient).

These advances in the diagnosis and treatment of autism spectrum disorders indicate the need for a new service delivery structure removed from large institutional bureaucracies, with siloed treatment areas and lines of reimbursement. We argue to replace that paradigm with an integrated, specialized medical home for neurodiverse individuals that provides multiple essential diagnostic and therapeutic services in one place and coordinates all the treatment for each patient. Such innovative healthcare service delivery models allow for novel and alternative reimbursement systems that can improve upon standard payment models. Present reimbursement is based upon payment for each individual and disparate procedure or treatment, thus incentivizing volume and siloed care delivery and discouraging long-term planning and the achievement of successful outcomes. We propose and are developing value-based alternative payment models that reward providers for achieving relevant outcomes tied to qualitative and quantitative patient improvements and outcomes, a win for all involved.

A COMPREHENSIVE CLINICAL MODEL FOR AUTISM

Although our clinical model is applicable to an array of neurological, neurodevelopmental, and neuropsychiatric disorders, autism is an excellent example of the value our approaches can provide. Tackling the multifaceted challenges of autism spectrum disorders requires a comprehensive clinical model for diagnosis, assessment, evaluation, and treatment. It is important for parents, family members, clinicians, insurers—indeed, everyone on the journey with the child in question—to understand the following for identifying potential therapeutic targets, ending "diagnostic journeys," and improving outcomes through the use of personalized and precision medicine techniques and modalities. What do a comprehensive clinical evaluation and assessment, neurodiagnostic and medical testing, and targeted therapeutic and treatment model look like?

CONSIDERATIONS OF ASSESSMENTS FOR CLINICAL PROFILING AND BIOLOGICAL SUB-PHENOTYPING FOR AUTISM SPECTRUM DISORDERS

▸ CLINICAL
  - Detailed Medical, Social, Psychiatric/Neurobehavioral, Educational, and Family History
    □ Review of Symptoms by Organ System
  - Comprehensive Examination
    □ Physical
    □ Neurological
    □ Neurodevelopmental
    □ Neuropsychiatric

▶ **BEHAVIORAL**
- Functional Behavior Analysis

▶ **NEUROPSYCHOLOGICAL**
- Evaluation and Testing

▶ **NEUROPHYSIOLOGICAL**
- Electroencephalography

▶ **NEUROGENOMIC**
- NextGen Sequencing/Whole Genome Sequencing

▶ **GASTROINTESTINAL**

▶ **IMMUNOLOGICAL**

▶ **NUTRITIONAL**

▶ **ENDOCRINOLOGICAL**

▶ **AUTONOMIC NERVOUS SYSTEM**

▶ **SLEEP-RELATED**

▶ **METABOLIC**

▶ **NEUROIMAGING**

▶ **OTHER**
- Urological
- Gynecological
- Bone Health
- Dermatological
- Cardiovascular
- Connective Tissue
- Visual Function
- Audiological

Clinical: As in many areas of medicine, the first step in a complete evaluation for a suspected or known case of ASD is an insightful and detailed medical history; presenting symptoms and complaints; pregnancy, birth, or neonatal complications or issues; past hospitalizations, surgeries, or significant medical illnesses, disorders, or diseases; identification of past head trauma or brain injury; past and present chronic drugs, medications, or supplements and any drug, medication, supplement, or other allergies; sleep history; vaccination history and complications; exposure to environmental toxins; inventory of development and behaviors; psychiatric history; educational history and review of learning issues; generational family history; description of social factors or family stressors; review of travel history; review of symptoms or issues by organ system, coupled with a comprehensive physical, neurological, neuropsychological, and neurodevelopmental examination and evaluation. This initial stage can provide clues to the biological underpinnings of autism spectrum disorders, inform about the next steps for neurodiagnostic testing and evaluations, and assess for comorbid or associated medical or systemic (other organ system) complications.

As information is gathered, there is a thought process concerning whether or not the patient is presenting with a process that is "acquired" (an event, exposure, or neurological insult to the developing brain occurring during fetal development or after birth, especially during younger years, when the brain is undergoing significant development and growth) or "predisposed" (genetically or otherwise); "static encephalopathy" (alterations of brain function or structure that is stable or improving at a slower rate than expected for a given age group), "dynamic/reversible encephalopathy" (chronic encephalopathy that has fluctuating trajectory as a response to therapies targeting pathophysiological processes outside of the brain), or "progressive/regressive encephalopathy" (loss of previously acquired developmental milestones or neurological function); "provoked" (identifiable trigger or instigator) or "unprovoked"; "focal" neurological or physical findings versus "diffuse/generalized" findings; and "acute" or "chronic" issues.

It is also important to be confident that the suspected diagnosis of autism is valid. Since autism is a "clinical" diagnosis—that is, there is no blood test, radiological study, or cognitive test that confirms an ASD diagnosis; rather, ASD is based on behaviors observed by third parties—there can be inaccuracies introduced into the diagnosis, especially at younger ages. There are standardized questionnaires and rating scales that can be used to validate the diagnosis and are often sufficient for obtaining insurance approval for ABA and other autism services. However, the current objective "gold standard" test is the Autism Diagnostic Observation Schedule-second edition (ADOS-2), requiring a trained and certified ADOS examiner who evokes and then observes and measures social interactions through various standardized tasks. ADOS is useful for determining the level and severity of autism but should be used in conjunction with other information to confirm an autism diagnosis. Technologies are being advanced to improve upon the ADOS by integrating the interplay of nervous system dynamics with social behaviors.[42]

Behavioral: Over the years extensive research has established the principles of applied behavior analysis (ABA) as a fundamental and empirically proven treatment modality for improving language, communication, and adaptive skills; improving attention, focus, social skills, memory, academics, and daily living skills; and decreasing problematic, harmful, or dangerous behaviors. Prior to implementing behavioral management, a "functional behavior analysis" is important

---

42 Harshit Bokadia et al., "Digitized ADOS: Social Interactions beyond the Limits of the Naked Eye," *Journal of Personalized Medicine* 10 (2020): 159, doi: 10.3390/jpm10040159.

for defining and quantifying maladaptive behaviors (severity, intensity, frequency), and to determine whether a problem behavior is being triggered or "reinforced" for a reason or environmental circumstance (garnering attention to the behavior [positive or negative], gaining access to preferred items or activity, attempting to escape from or avoid a demand or situation) or if the behavior is "automatically" reinforced, suggesting a biological activator.

ABA behavioral management is the process of systematically applying positive reinforcement strategies ("rewards") based upon the principles of behavior analysis to remove or reshape adverse reinforcers, improve socially significant behaviors to a meaningful degree, and demonstrate that the interventions employed are responsible for the improvement in behavior or skills through the collection of extensive data during therapy sessions. ABA is a very flexible treatment that can be adapted to the needs of each unique person, and can be delivered in office, at home, at school, and in community environments. ABA modalities are the agreed-upon standard of care due to empirical evidence supporting its efficacy in treating individuals of all ages with autism.

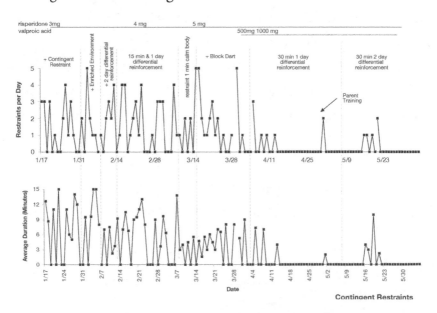

Graphically defining and quantifying maladaptive behaviors—a common methodology utilized by behavior analysts—can assist in guiding medical management. This is from an adolescent autistic patient I managed, at the time in a residential neurobehavioral stabilization unit. He required admission to this specialized unit because of very aggressive and other problematic behaviors, such as suddenly darting and running away to the point that staff had to physically restrain him for his and others' safety. The y axis displays the number of restraints per day and the average duration of each restraint, whereas the x axis is each day of data collection. Dotted vertical lines represent the noted behavioral management technique that was dropped in. On the top horizontal line are medication dosage changes. You can see from the graph that early on, despite increases to high doses of the neuroleptic medication risperidone along with different behavior management interventions, the frequency and intensity of the patient's maladaptive behaviors were relatively unchanged. So the behavior data is informing the medical team that the medication is ineffective. But once the antiseizure medication valproic acid was started, the problem behaviors diminished and essentially resolved. Again, the behavioral data help guide the medical team in using an effective medication. In this case, the response to an antiseizure medication does not mean the patient was having seizures but rather that certain antiseizure medications possess mood-stabilizing properties.

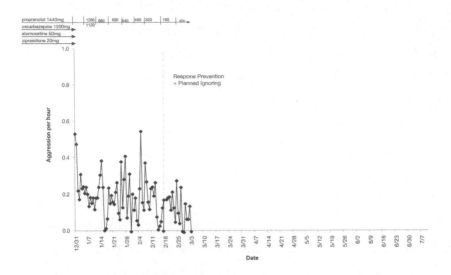

The figure above is another illustration of behavior data informing medical decision-making. When the patient was admitted to the neurobehavioral stabilization unit, he had been receiving a very complex medication regimen, including very high doses of the medication propranolol-a (beta-blocker) used for management of high blood pressure, which also can be used to temper autonomic over-responsivity and agitated behaviors. The initial medical plan was to simplify the patient's pharmacological regimen, starting with a slow wean of propranolol. As the medication dosage was reduced there was a concomitant reduction in aggressive behaviors. Thus, the behavior data reassured the medical team that propranolol was not a necessary medication for the patient, and in fact might have contributed to aggressive behaviors.

As an alternative to ABA, and sometimes in conjunction or combination with ABA, there is relation-based therapy (relationship development intervention, or RDI), often referred to as "floor time," as the interaction between the parent or therapist and child is done on the floor to interact "on their level." RDI involves engaging the child in games and activities they enjoy and following the child's lead to "expand their circles of communication."[43, 44, 45]

Neuropsychological: Neuropsychological evaluation and testing (i.e., the branch of psychology concerned with the physiological bases of psychological processes, and the relationship between brain-based functions such as language, memory, cognition, intellect, and emotions) can determine the degree of intellectual disability or cognitive impairment, characterize social deficits, and quantify communication deficits (language and social), even in minimally verbal children. Additionally, neuropsychological deficits can relate to neurophysiological changes, genetic variants, and abnormal laboratory testing. In other words, issues with a child's brain development can cause, or be caused by, physical changes in the brain, genetic abnormalities, and abnormal laboratory testing results that reflect problems in various physiological systems. Neuropsychological evaluation provides an important piece of a person's clinical profile and identification of potential treatment targets, as well as providing important objective, quantified, and standardized results for baseline and subsequent outcome measurements.

Neurophysiological: Epilepsy (recurrent seizures from abnormal electrical activity of the brain) is a major comorbid disorder in ASD, and ASD is a risk factor for the development of epilepsy. The burden of epilepsy in individuals with ASD has been reported to be as high

---

43   Stanley Greenspan and Serena Wieder, DIR®/Floortime™ model, The International Council on Developmental and Learning Disorders, 2008.

44   Jean Mercer, "Examining DIR/FloortimeTM as a Treatment for Children with Autism Spectrum Disorders: A Review of Research and Theory," *Research on Social Work Practice* 27, no. 5(2017): 625–635, https://doi.org/10.1177/1049731515583062.

45   Jessica Hobson et al., "The Relation between Severity of Autism and Caregiver-Child Interaction: A Study in the Context of Relationship Development Intervention," *Journal of Abnormal Child Psychology* 44 (2016): 745–755.

as 85 percent across the life span in those with autism spectrum disorders associated with intellectual disabilities. Electrical aberrations and abnormalities in specific parts of the brain are frequent in children with ASD with or without observable seizures. Language regression in autism can be caused by a form of epilepsy that may or may not have perceptible seizures (Landau-Kleffner syndrome, or electrical status epilepticus of sleep). Seizures can be subclinical, meaning that they are very subtle (staring for example) or brief and are not recognized by a caretaker. Clinical seizures can range from dramatic convulsions (severe muscular spasms with loss of consciousness) to sudden motor, sensory, or cognitive dysfunction with or without impairment of awareness or consciousness. In addition to the potential harm of recurrent or prolonged seizures, uncontrolled epilepsy can be associated with neuropsychological impairment or developmental regression. That is, children may suffer from a host of issues associated with autism that result from unseen seizures that are not captured by ordinary diagnostic tools. The device utilized to detect abnormal electrical activity of the brain, electroencephalography (EEG), may show seizurelike discharges ("spikes") without observable seizures "subclinical spikes" (also known as "interictal epileptiform discharges") that can be associated with cognitive impairment or behavioral aberrations, and such clinical symptoms may improve with antiepileptic drugs or other types of therapies that suppress the spikes.

Overall, since there is a very high incidence and prevalence of epilepsy, subclinical seizures, and subclinical spikes in autism spectrum disorders, EEG is an important assessment for many children and adults. Behavioral challenges for EEG acquisition can be overcome with behavioral desensitization and preparation with social stories, as well as the utilization of newer technologies such as high-density EEG

(HD-EEG) that employs a "sensor net" for the painless application of the head electrodes, as well as providing six times or more data and superior electrical source localization compared to conventional EEG.

HIGH-DENSITY ELECTROENCEPHALOGRAPHY (HD-EEG) "SENSOR NET"

- Sponge-based electrodes soaked in a solution of baby shampoo, warm water, and potassium chloride (KCl)
- No foul odors or glues/paste
- Rapid application (less than ten minutes), allowing for longer studies
- No scalp abrasion
- Reduced risk of infection
- Comfortable
- No pressure ulcer risk
- Improved compliance (no sedation or restraint)
- Whole head coverage and improved accuracy for epileptogenic source localization.

Neurogenomic: There is a genetic predisposition for most of the causes and complications of autism spectrum disorders. Understanding genomic relationships (i.e., the relationships among all of a person's genes and noncoding DNA) has revolutionized diagnosis and treatment of autism, not only by identifying new and novel biological mechanisms of autism spectrum disorders but also by eliminating unnecessary diagnostic testing and changing clinical management through improved diagnoses and identification of heretofore unknown treatment targets based on mechanisms of disease rather than symptom suppression. This reduces the reliance on ineffective therapies. Genomic relationships can also alert clinicians to potential problems in other organ systems. Next-generation sequencing (NGS or NextGen) of chromosomes, genes, and DNA is uncovering genetic variants that are capable of causing or contributing to more than 40 percent of autism spectrum disorder cases. This percentage continues to grow associated with the increasing prevalence of NGS testing and greater understanding of genetic factors influencing autism. This information is useful in heading off or ameliorating factors that exacerbate or complicate autism or that can end diagnostic journeys and avoid needless laboratory and invasive testing. In this way, neurogenomic evaluations and testing are extremely cost-effective and often change clinical management and improve outcomes.

Genomics is part of the concept of molecular profiling, but there are other "-omics" (OMICS) that are generating interest as important

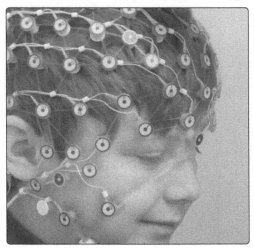

Sensor net

biomarkers for the diagnosis and clinical management of ASD: proteomics, metabolomics, transcriptomics, epigenetics, along with the molecular aspects of the gut microbiome and immune function. Genes are made up of DNA that has coding regions, and these coding regions will generate RNA that will eventually be synthesized into a protein. Proteins play various crucial roles throughout the body for structure (muscles, for example) and function (biochemical enzymes, for example). Pathological genetic variants will create defective proteins, and thus, can lead to various diseases and disorders, including ASD. The study of "proteomics" can provide information concerning underlying molecular issues with certain genes, may show a biomarker for altered or defective molecular processes, or can assist in determining whether treatments targeted at abnormal genetic mutations are useful. Moreover, certain parts of noncoding DNA outside of genes can regulate gene activity and expression, and certain types of RNA can regulate gene expression after the gene is transcribed. Genetic expression and function can also undergo epigenetic modification by various mechanisms, including methylation processes, other modifier genes, and an array of environmental exposures and influences. Epigenetics explains why two individuals can have the same pathological genetic variant but have different levels of severity or clinical manifestations.

Overall, these other OMICS areas require further study to better understand their translational power for screening, diagnosing, disease stratification, or assisting clinical management of ASD. Likely they will not be 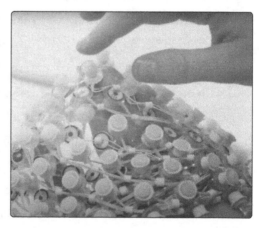 applicable to the broad spectrum of autism, but rather to biological subphenotypes. Nevertheless, the areas of genomics and other OMICS show great promise for a multimodal molecular/biological subphenotype or profile that is unique for an individual and can lead to precise and targeted therapies.

Gastrointestinal: Gastrointestinal (GI) disorders are often associated with ASDs, exacerbating underlying maladaptive behaviors, and hindering therapeutic progress. Identification and treatment of GI problems are essential to achieve success with other behavioral, medical, and nutritional therapeutic regimens. Additionally, microbiome imbalance (the community of microbes/bacteria within the human gut) can contribute to maladaptive behaviors in autism, and a growing body of research suggests that gut disorders may contribute to the development of autism itself. There are many treatments available for GI disorders, including anti-inflammatory and antimicrobial treatments, microbiota transfer therapy (fecal transplants), and various nutritional and nutraceutical products and supplements that can promote a balanced microbiome (the community of bacteria, fungi, viruses, and parasites that inhabit the gut in symbiotic coexistence).

Immunological: Immunological dysregulation can be found in ASD, including immune deficiencies, perturbations of innate immunity, autoimmunity, inflammation, and mast cell activation. Many individuals with ASD have identifiable immunologic abnormalities and disorders that can cause brain or systemic inflammation or be associated with opportunistic or chronic infections. Immunological disorders can often overlap with metabolic/mitochondrial disorders given that both processes rely upon cellular energy metabolism. Awareness of the influence of potentially treatable immunological dysfunction and the deleterious effects of infection or inflammation should trigger vigilance in identification of these factors in developing a clinical profile and biological treatment targets for children with ASD.

Nutritional: Children with ASDs often have inadequate dietary intake or gastrointestinal malabsorption, leading to protein, vitamin, and mineral deficiencies, which can further compound impairment of brain development or exacerbate underlying metabolic disorders. Additionally, certain pharmacological therapies can lead to nutritional or micronutrient deficiencies or disrupt the microbiome.

Endocrine: Dysfunction of the hypothalamic-pituitary-adrenal (HPA) axis affecting hormones such as thyroid, cortisol, and more may be causative or contributory to the pathogenesis ASD phenotypes, as well as contribute to maladaptive behavioral issues. Hormonal or gynecological changes or problems related to puberty can also contribute to behavioral difficulties. Endocrine disorders are often treatable. Appropriate identification and treatment of such disorders can contribute to improved outcomes.

Autonomic nervous system: Dysregulation of the autonomic nervous system (ANS, the neurological regulation of automatic responses to the environment, sometimes referred to as the fight-or-flight response) can exacerbate underlying maladaptive behavioral tendencies or be a complication of adjunctive pharmacological therapies. Clinicians treating ASD often overlook ANS over-responsivity and dysregulation, which in some instances can be related to treatable mitochondrial dysfunction and cellular ion channelopathies. Symptoms of mood disorder, anxiety, sensory over-responsiveness, violent behaviors, poor attention span, sleep disorders, and gastrointestinal dysfunction are among the frequent and treatable manifestations of autonomic dysfunction in ASDs.

Sleep-related: Sleep disorders and disturbances are very common in children with ASD. The prevalence of sleep disorders in ASD is extensive and includes obstructive sleep apnea, difficulty in settling to sleep, lengthy episodes of night waking with or without confusion, crying or screaming during sleep (sleep terror), bruxism (grinding teeth), nocturnal enuresis (bedwetting), REM sleep behavior disorder, early morning awakening, shortened night sleep, daytime sleepiness, and irregularities of the circadian rhythm. Sleep disorders are not only problematic for the patient, exacerbating daytime behavioral problems and impairing learning, but affect the entire family, upsetting their health and abilities as caretakers. Assessment of sleep patterns and hygiene is an essential component of the ASD clinical profile, often requiring further specific sleep tests (polysomnography) that can lead to medical, surgical, or behavioral interventions ameliorating these problems.

Metabolic: There is an array of disorders of cellular energy metabolism, mitochondrial disorders, and other metabolic derangements that can play a role in the development of autism and intellectual disabilities but particularly in mechanisms of biologically driven maladaptive behaviors and neuropsychiatric syndromes. Additionally, metabolic and mitochondrial disorders are increasingly recognized as causing or contributing to the development and maintenance of epilepsy, which is a common concomitant of ASD, and thus, epilepsy and ASD may share common pathophysiological origins. These disorders are often genetically predisposed but may require additional genetic or immunological mechanisms, or environmental influences to be triggered and cause harm. Similarly, these disorders may be prenatally or postnatally acquired from infection, inflammation, immunological mechanisms or exposure to environmental toxins. Historically, the diagnosis of metabolic disorders required extensive neuroradiological and laboratory investigations, some that are invasive (muscle biopsies, for example), but advances in genetics and genomics have found that many of these disorders and diseases can be identified initially with noninvasive genetic testing obviating the need for further testing, or at least pointing to very specific tests.

Neuroimaging: Neuroimaging—advanced imaging of the brain and central nervous system—should be considered when there are new or progressive abnormalities detected on clinical examination or evaluation, or focal or epileptiform patterns detected on EEG. Neuroimaging should also be considered in cases of ASD with epilepsy or other suspected brain diseases associated with autism (tuberous sclerosis, for example) or if there are clinical suspicions of diseases of the brain's vascular system or other structural brain abnormalities. Neuroimaging will often require sedation unless the patient can cooperate and lie still for the duration of the imaging, which has become shorter with advances in technology.

Other: There are other important organs and biological systems that require attention and vigilance for detecting abnormalities. Urological and gynecological health is often overlooked in those with ASD because of the difficulties patients have communicating such symptoms and the problems with examining sensitive areas in behaviorally challenged individuals. Bone health can be adversely affected by long-term pharmacological therapies. There are skin changes that provide potential clues about certain brain disorders. Congenital abnormalities of the heart can be associated with brain anomalies, and cardiac function can be adversely affected by various medications and metabolic, mitochondrial, or genetic disorders. Abnormalities of the connective tissue of the neuromuscular system (tendons, ligaments) can lead to hypermobility syndromes (joint laxity and excessive flexibility), which are increasingly recognized in association with ASD, and some rare subtypes can also cause arterial aneurysms.

Each of the above clinical and medical domains can lead the practitioner to appropriate and focused neurodiagnostic testing and eventually lead to targeted, precision therapies.

There are certain genetic disorders associated with ASD that can also increase the susceptibility toward the development of tumors and cancer, and thus, require ongoing surveillance. Eye health and visual function are important for overall functioning, and examination of the retina and optic nerve may also provide a window into potential brain diseases. Hearing is paramount for developing language, and formal audiological assessments are essential in those with language delays and impairments. And as with all individuals, those with ASD can develop many types of disorders and diseases unrelated to ASD but can often be overlooked because of communication impairments and behavioral challenges and barriers to examination.

These are the core concepts and procedures for our comprehensive clinical model that leads to personalized assessments, precision treatments, and improved outcomes: clinical profiling and biological phenotyping. Although the diagnosis of ASD can be established at the initial evaluation or soon thereafter prior to medical and laboratory testing, since ASD is a diagnosis that can be assigned without regard to its biological causes and contributions, the comprehensive clinical model provides clues and answers to the biological questions, and creates an overall road map for identifying precision treatment targets.

Not all patients require the complete array of the above investigations, but these clinical pathways lead to efficiencies and accuracies for further neurodiagnostic testing. For example, a neurogenomic evaluation may identify a genetic variant suggesting a high risk for a certain metabolic disorder, which then leads to a specific and focused laboratory test rather than extensive and expensive blood, urine, and invasive testing. Or a genetic variant that is considered highly pathogenic, affects brain development and structure, and is the molecular cause of the child's autism will suggest there is no need to go down the path of extensive laboratory or invasive testing. Each of the above clinical and medical domains can lead the practitioner to appropriate and focused neurodiagnostic testing and eventually lead to targeted, precision therapies.

The other important aspect of our clinical model is the combination of access and continuity of transdisciplinary specialized care associated with qualitative and quantitative objective and analytical data, allowing for continual monitoring and reassessment of provided clinical management. Thus, we can adjust therapies and interventions if progress plateaus or regresses, or if goals or expectations are not met. This ability to reexamine, reevaluate, and reconsider leads to optimized outcomes.

SPECIALTY CARE MEDICAL HOME IS THE BEST MODEL

Thus, autism is so much more than a disorder, or even a spectrum of disorders; it is a wide-ranging array of physical, medical, neurological, developmental, and psychological conditions and disorders, often accompanied by a multitude of complicating factors. Assessing and treating ASD requires the significant expertise of a team of providers focused singularly on each individual patient and their family. People with ASD may share common traits, but each person is unique.

For many individuals and their families dealing with the challenges of autism, their long and frustrating diagnostic journey is beginning to come to an end, with a hope for improved outcomes and quality of life. More than anything, it is this never-ending hope that keeps families dealing with the scourges of autism battling through their many challenges to better outcomes for their child and all those around them.

The merging of an innovative healthcare delivery system for special needs populations, Specialty Care Medical Home, with an integrated and transdisciplinary/multidisciplinary clinical model, is the formula for improved outcomes and a healthier, happier, more independent life for individuals with ASD and their families: improved diagnoses based on recognition of innumerable facets and comorbidities associated with the condition, clinical pathways for pragmatic and efficacious neurodiagnostic testing and evaluations, and personalized and customized multimodal therapies based on the acknowledgment that each individual experiences ASD differently.

As I reflect on where we started and how far we have come, after over thirty years of clinical experience working with special needs populations and their families, and over fifteen years developing and refining our clinical model and innovative Specialty Care Medical Home integrated healthcare delivery system, I strongly believe that we and other like-minded organizations can achieve a revolution in the care of ASD and related disorders. We have demonstrated the ability to help patients and families improve their quality of life, become healthier, achieve success, live a more independent life, and have enhanced inclusion into society. Special needs populations, and ASD in particular, are expanding in pandemic proportions. Thus, there is an urgency for innovative healthcare models that provide value and address the wants, needs, essentials, and requirements of individuals with ASD, their families and caretakers, healthcare providers, educational systems, residential systems, and payers (government and commercial insurances, employers, other).

This has been my mission and journey. I am forever grateful for the tens of thousands of patients and families who have allowed me, my professional colleagues, administrators, and staff members to help them along their difficult path and odyssey. They are the true heroes of this story—thrust into a world of challenges and struggles that they could never have imagined, through no fault of their own but solely because of random quirks of nature or unforeseeable life events. Yet they have embraced their destiny with determination, tenacity, aplomb, selflessness, courage, and grace on a daily basis, sacrificing their own needs for the betterment of their kin. Their trials, tribulations, and insights have provided my inspiration and motivation for taking risks to develop better systems of care.

Adversity provides life lessons and can make us wiser and stronger. Suffering can evolve into achievement and success. As anyone who has had the opportunity to share time with individuals who have special needs can attest, these children and adults have much to offer and teach us all. Stan Adams Jr. is one such example. I have known Stan and his family for many years and have been fortunate to have played a part in his and his mother's, Karyn's, journey. Stan has had to overcome obstacles of autism, mild intellectual disability, expressive-receptive language disorder, autonomic over-responsivity, clinical and subclinical epilepsy, dyspraxia (problems with coordination), congenital heart defect, non-celiac gluten sensitivity, and anxiety and other neuropsychiatric symptoms. But with a supportive and loving family, which has not allowed him to be defined purely by his diagnoses but rather by focusing on his abilities and not his disabilities, along with his own internal drives that we cannot fully fathom, Stan has developed into a fine young adult with an array of accomplishments, including small steps such as learning how to ride a bicycle, larger strides to employment at a local food establishment, and amazing triumphs of developing into a competitive swimmer and being voted prom king and Distinguished Male Athlete of the Year for his high school.

It is my desire for this book to provide hope and reassurance to individuals, families, and caretakers struggling with adversity that there are many alternative approaches presently available—lights at the end of the tunnel for better days ahead. I have described many gaps in our healthcare system and proposed transformative healthcare delivery remedies for an oft-neglected segment of society—those with special needs. I hope that our approaches for disruptive innovation have contributed to the betterment of life for those individuals with special needs and their families. And there is much to look forward to, as we continue to learn and understand the biological complexities and intricacies that cause neurological disorders and neurodevelopmental disabilities and experience rapid advancements in various technologies, from genomics to artificial intelligence and much more, all contributing to better tools for diagnosis and novel and efficacious treatments, leading to even better and brighter optimized outcomes.

This book can be summed up by the title of Karyn Adams's recent book about her son Stan's life story: *Don't Give Up*. And to paraphrase biblical scripture, "If you make a difference in one life, you make a difference in the whole world."

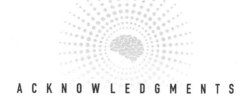

ACKNOWLEDGMENTS

I am immensely grateful to my beloved wife, Dr. Pnina Mintz, for her unwavering support, love, and guidance throughout our journey together. She provided the strength, courage, and inspiration for taking on the risk of cofounding NeurAbilities Healthcare, and we have not looked back.

I am deeply appreciative for our three (now adult) children, Matan, Magen, and Maya, for their incredible understanding of their parents' job demands and responsibilities. During their school breaks and transitions, they also gained invaluable work experiences and learned the importance of service to others. In particular, Matan stayed on and became a key contributor to NeurAbilities Healthcare's growth and development as digital marketing strategist and chief designer, transforming the digital presence and overall brand of NeurAbilities.

I am overwhelmed with gratitude for the many incredible staff, employees, clinicians, consultants, advisors, volunteers, students, and trainees who have each played a significant role and factor in the growth and development of NeurAbilities Healthcare. From front desk to back office, direct care to support staff, managers to executive management, technicians to technical support, receptionists to digital communications, schedulers to hope ambassadors, accountants to billers, recruiters to credentialing, IT to operations, marketing to community relations—no role is too small or inconsequential. We are the sum of our parts.

It has been an honor to have engaged and collaborated with so many dedicated physicians, nurses, medical assistants, neuropsychologists, psychologists, therapists, behavior analysts, and other direct care and professional staff who have made a difference in the lives of so many patients and their families.

I am forever thankful for the support from the many persons and families we have had the privilege to serve. It is your courage in the face of adversity that provides daily inspiration and validation for our vision and mission. I would like to extend special thanks to the families who have inspired and shared their stories and experiences with me throughout this writing journey so that others may benefit.

I am immensely appreciative of the confidence Council Capital has had in our vision and mission, and because of their support, we have been able to bring our ideas for improved healthcare delivery models to a higher level and broader audience. Along with this support has been the creation of a new and highly skilled executive management team, led by CEO Kathleen Stengel, who will be leading us to even brighter horizons.

Special thanks to Sandra Lewis for her invaluable assistance with the many tasks necessary for completing the book, and to Barry Waldman and Lauren Steffes from Advantage|Forbes Books for their encouragement, assistance, and technical input throughout the writing process.

Finally, I am humbled by the many teachers, mentors, colleagues, students, and trainees whom I have had the opportunity to learn from over the years.

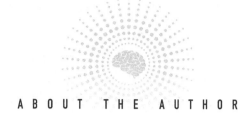

MARK MINTZ, MD, is chief medical officer and founder of NeurAbilities Healthcare and the Clinical Research Center of New Jersey (CRCNJ). Dr. Mintz is quadruple board certified in neurology (with special qualification in child neurology), neurodevelopmental disabilities, epilepsy, and pediatrics. Dr. Mintz is or has been a member of the faculties of the Rutgers-New Jersey Medical School, University of Pennsylvania School of Medicine, and Cooper Medical School of Rowan University.

Dr. Mintz is widely published in medical literature, is on the editorial boards of peer-reviewed journals, and has been an invited lecturer at a large number of national and international conferences. In addition to functioning as the principal investigator on a variety of clinical research studies, Dr. Mintz has participated on an array of committees, task forces, and research projects of the National Institutes of Health, American Academy of Neurology, American Academy of Pediatrics, Child Neurology Society, and the New Jersey Governor's Office. Dr. Mintz has been an advocate for transforming healthcare delivery systems for special needs populations, which has led to the creation of the innovative and unique Specialty Care Medical Home model utilized at NeurAbilities Healthcare.

Additionally, Dr. Mintz has served in the National Health Service Corps of the US Public Health Service and has volunteered for medical relief missions in Romania and Russia. Dr. Mintz's clinical and research interests include neurodevelopmental and intellectual disabilities, autism spectrum disorders, epilepsy, neuropsychiatric disorders, brain injury/concussions, ADHD, learning disorders, Tourette's/tic disorders, genetic and metabolic disorders, and NeuroAIDS.

ABOUT NEURABILITIES HEALTHCARE

NEURABILITIES HEALTHCARE was born from a vision to bring experts of neurological, developmental, cognitive, and behavioral care together within the same organization, working collaboratively to provide a seamless experience for patients. Our medical and clinical evaluation teams produce informed diagnoses and personalized therapeutic treatment recommendations. Our transdisciplinary team of neurologists, developmental-behavioral pediatricians, advanced practice nurses, neuropsychologists, neurotechnologists, therapists, and behavior analysts take both a curious and investigative approach to learn about the whole patient, assimilating our core values of compassion, collaboration, integrity, excellence, and joy. Our unique, innovative, and seminal Specialty Care Medical Home model of healthcare delivery for special needs populations is the foundation of a place where patients can feel cared for and heard. NeurAbilities Healthcare impacts the lives of individuals looking to find answers, solutions, and optimized outcomes.

To learn more about services provided at NeurAbilities or to subscribe to the NeurAbilities newsletter for regular updates, visit www.NeurAbilities.com.

To learn more about Dr. Mark Mintz or to submit a contact request, visit https://neurabilities.com/our-team/staff-bio-mark-mintz-md/.

TO FOLLOW NEURABILITIES ON SOCIAL MEDIA:
facebook.com/NeurAbilities
Instagram.com/NeurAbilities_Healthcare
Linkedin.com/company/NeurAbilities

Printed in the USA
CPSIA information can be obtained
at www.ICGtesting.com
JSHW022341140824
68134JS00019B/1616